Implantable Auditory Devices

Editors

DARIUS KOHAN
SUJANA S. CHANDRASEKHAR

OTOLARYNGOLOGIC CLINICS OF NORTH AMERICA

www.oto.theclinics.com

Consulting Editor
SUJANA S. CHANDRASEKHAR

April 2019 • Volume 52 • Number 2

ELSEVIER

1600 John F. Kennedy Boulevard • Suite 1800 • Philadelphia, Pennsylvania, 19103-2899

http://www.oto.theclinics.com

OTOLARYNGOLOGIC CLINICS OF NORTH AMERICA Volume 52, Number 2
April 2019 ISSN 0030-6665, ISBN-13: 978-0-323-67817-9

Editor: Jessica McCool
Developmental Editor: Sara Watkins

Otolaryngologic Clinics of North America (ISSN 0030-6665) is published bimonthly by Elsevier, Inc., 360 Park Avenue South, New York, NY 10010-1710. Months of issue are February, April, June, August, October, and December. Business and Editorial Offices: 1600 John F. Kennedy Blvd., Suite 1800, Philadelphia, PA 19103-2899. Customer Service Office: 6277 Sea Harbor Drive, Orlando, FL 32887-4800. Periodicals postage paid at New York, NY and additional mailing offices. Subscription prices are $412.00 per year (US individuals), $889.00 per year (US institutions), $100.00 per year (US student/resident), $548.00 per year (Canadian individuals), $1127.00 per year (Canadian institutions), $564.00 per year (international individuals), $1127.00 per year (international institutions), $270.00 per year (international & Canadian student/resident). Foreign air speed delivery is included in all *Clinics'* subscription prices. All prices are subject to change without notice. **POSTMASTER:** Send address changes to *Otolaryngologic Clinics of North America*, Elsevier Health Sciences Division, Subscription Customer Service, 3251 Riverport Lane, Maryland Heights, MO 63043. **Telephone: 1-800-654-2452 (U.S. and Canada); 314-447-8871 (outside U.S. and Canada). Fax: 314-447-8029. E-mail: journalscustomerservice-usa@elsevier.com (for print support); journalsonlinesupport-usa@elsevier.com (for online support).**

Reprints. For copies of 100 or more of articles in this publication, please contact the Commercial Reprints Department, Elsevier Inc., 360 Park Avenue South, New York, NY 10010-1710. Tel.: 212-633-3874; Fax: 212-633-3820; E-mail: reprints@elsevier.com.

Otolaryngologic Clinics of North America is also published in Spanish by McGraw-Hill Interamericana Editores S.A., P.O. Box 5-237, 06500 Mexico D.F., Mexico.

Otolaryngologic Clinics of North America is covered in *MEDLINE/PubMed (Index Medicus), Current Contents/Clinical Medicine, Excerpta Medica, BIOSIS, Science Citation Index,* and *ISI/BIOMED.*

Contributors

CONSULTING EDITOR

SUJANA S. CHANDRASEKHAR, MD
Partner, ENT and Allergy Associates, LLP, Past President, American Academy of Otolaryngology-Head and Neck Surgery, Clinical Professor of Otolaryngology, Zucker School of Medicine at Hofstra-Northwell, Hempstead, New York; Clinical Associate Professor of Otolaryngology, Icahn School of Medicine at Mount Sinai, New York, New York, USA

EDITORS

DARIUS KOHAN, MD
Director of Otology/Neurotology, Lenox Hill Hospital/Manhattan Eye Ear Nose Throat Hospital-Northwell Health System, Clinical Associate Professor, Department of Otolaryngology, NYU School of Medicine, New York, New York, USA

SUJANA S. CHANDRASEKHAR, MD
Partner, ENT and Allergy Associates, LLP, Past President, American Academy of Otolaryngology-Head and Neck Surgery, Clinical Professor of Otolaryngology, Zucker School of Medicine at Hofstra-Northwell, Hempstead, New York; Clinical Associate Professor of Otolaryngology, Icahn School of Medicine at Mount Sinai, New York, New York, USA

AUTHORS

MANOHAR LAL BANCE, MB ChB, MSc, FRCSC, FRCS
Otology and Skull Base Unit, Cambridge University Hospitals NHS Foundation Trust, Hills Road, Cambridge, United Kingdom

SELENA E. BRIGGS, MD, PhD, MBA, MAUML, FACS
Vice Chair, Department of Otolaryngology, MedStar Washington Hospital Center, Associate Professor, Department of Otolaryngology, Georgetown University Medical Center, Washington, DC, USA

C.Y. JOSEPH CHANG, MD
Director, Texas Ear Center, Clinical Professor, Department of Otorhinolaryngology–Head and Neck Surgery, University of Texas McGovern Medical School, Houston, Texas, USA

BAISHAKHI CHOUDHURY, MD
Assistant Professor, Department of Otolaryngology Head and Neck Surgery, Loma Linda University Health, Redlands, California, USA

MARC D'APRILE, ScD, CCC-A
Director of Audiology, New York Otolaryngology Group, New York, New York, USA

JULIE DAUGHERTY, PhD, NP-C
Assistant Director of Research for the Ear Research Foundation, Silverstein Institute, Sarasota, Florida, USA

SOHA N. GHOSSAINI, MD
Otology-Neurotology, Ear Nose and Throat Associates of New York, Auburndale, New York, USA

TYLER A. JANZ, BS
University of Central Florida College of Medicine, Orlando, Florida, USA

DANIEL JETHANAMEST, MD
Assistant Professor, Director, Division of Otology and Neurotology, Department of Otolaryngology–Head and Neck Surgery, NYU Langone Health, New York, New York, USA

ANA H. KIM, MD
Associate Professor, Medical Director, Cochlear Implant Program, Department of Otolaryngology, Columbia University Medical Center, New York, New York, USA

DARIUS KOHAN, MD
Director of Otology/Neurotology, Lenox Hill Hospital/Manhattan Eye Ear Nose Throat Hospital-Northwell Health System, Clinical Associate Professor, Department of Otolaryngology, NYU School of Medicine, New York, New York, USA

MEGAN KUHLMEY, AuD
Assistant Professor, Audiology Director, Cochlear Implant Program, Department of Otolaryngology, Columbia University Medical Center, New York, New York, USA

JENNIFER WING YEE LEE, BSc(Med), MBBS, MS, FRACS
Otology and Skull Base Unit, Cambridge University Hospitals NHS Foundation Trust, Hills Road, Cambridge, United Kingdom

SARA LERNER, AuD
ENT and Allergy Associates, New York, New York, USA

CAROL LI, MD
Otolaryngology Resident, Department of Otolaryngology, Columbia University Medical Center, New York, New York, USA

JENNIFER MAW, MD, FRCS(C)
Adjunct Clinical Associate Professor, Department of Otolaryngology Head and Neck Surgery, Stanford University, Stanford, California; President, Ear Associates and Rehabilitation Services, Inc, San Jose, California, USA

MIA E. MILLER, MD
House Clinic, Los Angeles, California, USA

ASHLEY M. NASSIRI, MD, MBA
Resident Physician, The Otology Group of Vanderbilt, Department of Otolaryngology–Head and Neck Surgery, Vanderbilt University Medical Center, Nashville, Tennessee, USA

DIEGO A. PRECIADO, MD, PhD
Division of Pediatric Otolaryngology, Children's National Health System, Professor of Surgery, Pediatrics, and Genomics and Precision Medicine, George Washington University School of Medicine, Washington, DC, USA

BRIAN K. REILLY, MD
Division of Pediatric Otolaryngology, Children's National Health System, George
Washington University School of Medicine, Washington, DC, USA

ROBERT M. RHODES, MD
Resident Physician, The Department of Otolaryngology Head and Neck Surgery,
The University of Oklahoma Health Sciences Center, Oklahoma City, Oklahoma,
USA

ALEJANDRO RIVAS, MD
Associate Professor, The Otology Group of Vanderbilt, Department of Otolaryngology–
Head and Neck Surgery, Vanderbilt University Medical Center, Nashville, Tennessee,
USA

PAMELA C. ROEHM, MD, PhD
Department of Otolaryngology–Head and Neck Surgery, Temple University School of
Medicine, Philadelphia, Pennsylvania, USA

MICHAEL D. SEIDMAN, MD, FACS
Director, Otologic/Neurotologic/Skull Base Surgery, Medical Director Wellness and
Integrative Medicine, Advent Health (Celebration and South Campuses); Professor,
Otolaryngology Head & Neck Surgery, University of Central Florida, Orlando, Florida;
Adjunct Professor, Otolaryngology Head & Neck Surgery, University of South Florida,
Tampa, Florida, USA

JACK A. SHOHET, MD
Shohet Ear Associates, Orange County, Newport Beach, California; Clinical Professor,
Otolaryngology Head and Neck Surgery, University of California, Irvine, California,
USA

JOSHUA SMITH, DO
Clinical Fellow, Otology, Silverstein Institute, Sarasota, Florida, USA

NEIL M. SPERLING, MD
New York Otolaryngology Group, Affiliate Assistant Professor of Clinical Otolaryngology,
Weill Cornell Medical College, New York, New York; Adjunct Associate Professor of
Otolaryngology, SUNY Downstate College of Medicine, Brooklyn, New York, USA

MAJA SVRAKIC, MD, MSEd
Department of Otolaryngology, Long Island Jewish Medical Center, Hearing and Speech
Center, Northwell Health, New Hyde Park, New York, USA

BETTY S. TSAI DO, MD, FACS
Associate Professor, The Department of Otolaryngology Head and Neck Surgery,
The University of Oklahoma Health Sciences Center, Oklahoma City, Oklahoma,
USA

ANDREA VAMBUTAS, MD
Department of Otolaryngology, Long Island Jewish Medical Center, Hearing and Speech
Center, Northwell Health, New Hyde Park, New York, USA

JACK WAZEN, MD, FACS
Chairman, Department of Surgery, Past Chair, Division of Otolaryngology Head and
Neck Surgery, Sarasota Memorial Hospital, Vice President, Director of Research of the
Silverstein Institute, Silverstein Institute, Sarasota, Florida, USA

JENNIFER R. WHITE, MD
Resident Physician, Department of Otolaryngology, Medstar Georgetown University Hospital, Washington, DC, USA

ROBERT J. YAWN, MD
Neurotology Fellow, The Otology Group of Vanderbilt, Department of Otolaryngology–Head and Neck Surgery, Vanderbilt University Medical Center, Nashville, Tennessee, USA

SCOTT E. YERDON, AuD, F-AAA
Staff Audiologist, New York Otolaryngology Group, New York, New York, USA

Contents

> Implantable auditory devices (IADs) are a viable hearing restoration option for patients with hearing loss. Conditions such as chronic otitis externa, congenital aural atresia, and chronic otitis media can be treated with a variety of implants. Progressive disease are also amenable to restoration with IADs, providing stabilized hearing. When considering the best rehabilitative options, the patient's preference, ease of surgery, ease of device use, quality of life, and the traditional alternatives (such as ossiculoplasty, hearing aids, and cochlear implants) need to be considered. Patients with conductive, mixed, and sensorineural losses, mild to severe in nature, can be candidates for IADs.

> This article examines and evaluates methods, from an audiologist's perspective, of reducing common complaints with conventional hearing aids and issues such as the occlusion effect, acoustic feedback, discomfort, and insufficient gain. Although often successful, reducing one problem may have the tradeoff of causing another issue. This article is meant to provide information to the reader regarding modern conventional hearing aids, the means to alleviate common problems in the clinic, and when middle ear implants and osseointegrated implants can be beneficial.

 Video content accompanies this article at http://www.oto.theclinics.com.

> A new category of hearing technology has emerged that comprises devices inserted deep into the ear canal. Although not implanted, they represent an extension of what is expected of a traditional hearing aid. There are advantages to these devices, but they are not suited for all individuals with hearing loss. This category consists of 2 devices currently available in the

Bone conduction implant devices rely on osseointegration of titanium implants with the underlying skull, characterized by endosseous healing and de-novo bone formation both surrounding and onto the implant surface. The key steps in osseointegration are the initial tissue response to implantation, peri-implant osteogenesis, and peri-implant bone remodeling. There is increasing evidence that osseointegration is primarily an immune-mediated process with the key players being the complement cascade and macrophages, which form part of the host innate immunity. Implant design and composition, patient systemic factors, surgical technique, and loading characteristics can all affect the success of osseointegration.

Osseointegrated auditory devices (OADs) are hearing devices that use an external receiver/processor that stimulates bone conduction of sound via a titanium prosthesis that is drilled into the bone of the cranium. Since their introduction in 1977, OADs have undergone substantial evolution, including changes in manufacturing of the implant, improvements in the external sound processor, and simplification of implantation techniques. Expansion of criteria for patient candidacy for implantation has occurred corresponding with changes in the implants and processors.

Percutaneous osseointegrated bone conduction auditory devices provide excellent auditory rehabilitation. Device-related complications relate to skin abutment interface and cosmetic concerns, resulting in the development of transcutaneous devices. The Sophono and Baha Attract are safe and considered cosmetically superior to the percutaneous Baha Connect and Ponto. They provide excellent auditory enhancement; however, owing to indirect connectivity between processor and implant, there is on average 5- to 7-db less gain when compared with percutaneous bone-anchored implants. Surgical implantation of either device is usually performed under monitored sedation, in an ambulatory setting, with less than a 1-hour operative time, and minimal complications.

Bonebridge is an active bone conduction device that consists of a bone conduction-floating mass transducer (BC-FMT) and magnet internally and an audio processor externally. Surgery for implantation can be performed under local anesthesia but requires surgical planning for adequate bone depth for the BC-FMT well. Bonebridge does not require osseointegration to function, so the device can be activated early. One disadvantage of Bonebridge is the sizable artifact on MRI created by the internal magnet. Studies of Bonebridge implantation demonstrate few complications, and hearing outcomes are audiologically equivalent to other bone conduction devices.

Active auditory implants, such as the Maxum, provide significantly improved hearing function compared to hearing aids in patients with moderate to severe hearing loss who are not reaching their cochlear hearing potential. The speech perception gap (SPG), defined as PB Max (phonetically balanced maximum) minus word recognition score with hearing aid, is a useful measure of inadequate hearing aid performance. The Maxum middle ear implant provides significantly improved performance over hearing aids in patients with significant SPG because of superior high frequency gain. Patients with PB Max 60% or greater with SPG are possible candidates for the implant.

The Vibrant Soundbridge is a semi-implantable, active middle ear implant that is a safe and effective treatment for patients with sensorineural hearing loss. Since Food and Drug Administration approval for this indication, many international investigators have expanded its use for conductive and mixed hearing losses. This article reviews the author's experience and the international uses of this versatile device.

The Envoy Esteem and the Carina system are the 2 totally implantable hearing devices. The Esteem is designed for patients with bilateral moderate to severe sensorineural hearing loss who have an unaided speech discrimination score of greater than and equal to 40%. The Carina system is designed for patients with moderate to severe sensorineural hearing loss or those with mixed hearing loss. The Esteem offers a technologically advanced method to provide improvements in hearing and is available in the United States, whereas the Carina system is currently not available in the United States.

Electric acoustic stimulation (EAS), also known as hybrid stimulation, is indicated for individuals with intact low-frequency hearing and profound high-frequency hearing loss. Although low frequencies contribute to speech perception, these individuals are usually only able to detect vowels, but few or no consonants, and thus have difficulty with word understanding and hearing in noise. EAS uses the cochlear implant electrode array to stimulate the high frequencies within the basal turn of the cochlea coupled with a hearing aid to convey the low frequencies at the apical turn in the same ear.

Hearing loss in the pediatric population can have significant social and developmental implications. Early auditory rehabilitation by at least 6 months of age is imperative. Although traditional hearing aids are often a first-line treatment option, there is a wide array of implantable auditory devices available. This article describes the indications for such devices as they pertain to the pediatric population, including osseointegrated bone-conduction devices, middle ear implants, cochlear implants, and auditory brainstem implants.

Hearing loss is common in the geriatric population. Most hearing loss is associated with presbycusis or age-related hearing loss, impacting one-third of individuals over 65 years and increasing in prevalence with age. Hearing loss impacts quality of life, psychological health, and cognition. Implantable auditory devices are an exceptional option to improve hearing and quality of life. Various implantable auditory devices have been implemented safely with significant improvement in communication and performance on auditory tasks. Counseling is essential to establishing realistic expectations. Rehabilitation may be required to optimize outcomes and auditory performance with use.

Children with hearing loss and additional disabilities can benefit from cochlear implants and other implantable auditory devices. Although each individual child must be evaluated, and families uniquely counseled on goals and realistic expectations, overall many gains and benefits are possible in this population. In this article, an overview of the considerations for this group is discussed and outcomes are reviewed, including auditory and speech measures as well as benefits in other skills and quality of life.

Auditory neuropathy spectrum disorder (ANSD) is a complex and heterogeneous disorder associated with altered neural synchrony with respect to auditory stimuli. Patients have characteristic auditory findings including normal otoacoustic emissions in the setting of abnormal auditory brainstem response. Patients with ANSD have a high incidence of comorbid developmental delay that may impact speech outcomes. Treatment options for ANSD include hearing amplification and cochlear implantation. The article highlights issues and controversies with the diagnosis and treatment of this complex disorder.

Hearing rehabilitation has been recognized as a crucial tool to maintain communicative and social skills. The availability of hearing aids and auditory implants ought not be limited to the wealthy and to those who can afford them. Multidisciplinary efforts in reducing costs are necessary and include reduction of the item costs, insurance coverage, and the ability to perform certain procedures in an office setting, eliminating hospital and facilities fees and anesthesia bills.

The advances in technology leading to rapid developments in implantable auditory devices are constantly evolving. Devices are becoming smaller, less visible, and more efficient. The ability to preserve hearing outcomes with cochlear implantation will continue to evolve as surgical techniques improve with the use of continuous feedback during the procedure as well as with intraoperative delivery of drugs and robot assistance. As engineering methods improve, there may one day be a totally implantable aid that is self-sustaining in hearing-impaired patients making them indistinguishable from patients without hearing loss.

OTOLARYNGOLOGIC CLINICS
OF NORTH AMERICA

THE CLINICS ARE AVAILABLE ONLINE!
Access your subscription at:
www.theclinics.com

Foreword

Bridging the Sizeable Gap Between Hearing Aids and Cochlear Implants

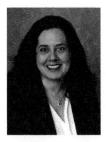

Sujana S. Chandrasekhar, MD
Consulting Editor

The first form of hearing assistance, still in use today, is cupping the hand behind the pinna. It adds about 8 dB, primarily in the frequency range of 1.6 to 2 kHz.[1] The first hearing aids were described in the seventeenth century and were the long trumpets used by sailors to hear the voices of other sailors calling to them over long distances at sea. These devices were tailored to civilian life and sold as ear trumpets or cornets, many of which were decorated beautifully to match the user's outfits. Commercial development of these devices was first reported in 1800 by the FC Rein Company, which also sold hearing fans and speaking tubes, able to amplify sound, but bulky and not portable. In 1819, the company made a hearing throne for the ailing King John VI of Portugal.[2] Toward the end of that century, invisibility became more sought after, with "acoustic headbands" and the like, as form beat out functionality. After the inventions of the telephone and the microphone, the first electronic hearing aids were built in the 1870s and onward. These, of course, got smaller and better in terms of amplification and sound clarity. We continue to see huge advances in conventional hearing aid technology, enabling wider utilization and better patient satisfaction.

Meanwhile, after Alessandro Volta first stimulated his own inner ear with electrical current in 1800, in 1957, André Djourno and Charles Eyriès tried to stimulate the facial nerve in a patient with extensive bilateral cholesteatoma with an electrical current. The face did not move but the patient experienced auditory sensations. In 1961, William House and John Doyle (US) placed a single-channel electrode through the round window in two patients, resulting in auditory perception. In 1967, Graeme Clarke (Australia) began experiments with multielectrode auditory implants in animals. Single-channel, and then multichannel, cochlear implants have been commercially available since 1972.[3] Initially approved only for bilaterally profound postlingually deafened

Otolaryngol Clin N Am 52 (2019) xiii–xiv
https://doi.org/10.1016/j.otc.2018.11.019

adults, they are now approved for moderately severe to profound sensorineural hearing loss, in unilateral cases, and in children.

But what about the patients for whom conventional hearing aids are not enough, but cochlear implants are too much? In this issue of *Otolaryngologic Clinics of North America*, I had the great good fortune of working once again with my former senior resident and current colleague, Dr Darius Kohan, to explore the realm of implantable hearing technology. The issue is organized along the lines of an excellent implantable auditory devices (IAD) conference that was Darius' brainchild and that has been presented in whole and in part in New York City and at the American Academy of Otolaryngology–Head and Neck Surgery Annual Meeting.

The authors of each article in this issue of *Otolaryngologic Clinics of North America* contribute valuable information as to how to assess patients and think about IADs. These articles cover the limitations of conventional hearing aids and indications for IADs, the physiology and application details of osseointegration in IADs, and the coupling of devices to the ossicles or round window. As mentioned above, solving a hearing dilemma is almost always followed by patient request for cosmesis, invisibility, and desire for more. This is seen in the discussions of totally implantable devices as well as electroacoustic stimulation. There are special populations for whom attention and consideration must be given; each of these is addressed comprehensively by the authors of those articles. Financial considerations are important, and the current situation in the United States is detailed. Finally, our patients ask us what is to come, and if they would be "burning bridges" by having an implant now rather than waiting. The last article articulates the future as it is currently known.

I always enjoy working with the Guest Editors on each issue of *Otolaryngologic Clinics of North America*. This time around, I got to be a co-Guest Editor and wear a couple of hats. I hope that you, the reader, enjoy the articles in this issue and find them to be helpful as you counsel patients with hearing loss and their families.

Sujana S. Chandrasekhar, MD
ENT and Allergy Associates, LLP
18 East 48th Street, 2nd Floor
New York, NY 10017, USA

E-mail address:
ssc@nyotology.com

REFERENCES

1. Barr-Hamilton RM. The cupped hand as an aid to hearing. Br J Audiol 1983;17(1): 27–30.
2. Concealed hearing devices of the 18th century, Bernard Becker Medical Library, Washington University School of Medicine, St Louis, MO. Available at: http://beckerexhibits.wustl.edu/did/19thcent/index.htm. Accessed November 23, 2018.
3. Hainarosie M, Zainea V, Hainarosie R. The evolution of cochlear implant technology and its clinical relevance [special issue 2]. J Med Life 2014;7(Spec No. 2):1–4.

Preface

Implantable Auditory Devices: Bridging the Gap Between Conventional Hearing Aids and Cochlear Implants

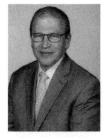

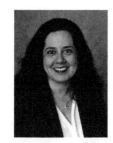

Darius Kohan, MD   Sujana S. Chandrasekhar, MD
Editors

Technology for managing hearing loss is rapidly evolving, regardless of whether patients have a sensorineural, conductive, or mixed auditory deficit. Modalities applicable for hearing loss range from mild to profound. Otolaryngologists are relatively comfortable with the concepts behind conventional hearing aids and cochlear implants. However, the options for hearing losses that cannot be appropriately fit with either of these are expanding, and the technological advances are remarkable. The focus of this issue of *Otolaryngologic Clinics of North America* is on implantable auditory devices: active middle ear implants and osseointegrated options for aural rehabilitation.

The invited contributing authors are distinguished leaders in their field specializing in the topic of their article. The medical and audiologic indications for different aural rehabilitation options are discussed in detail, including deep fitting canal devices, percutaneous and transcutaneous osseointegrated devices, active ossicle coupling devices, and totally implantable auditory processors. Pediatric patients, geriatric patients, and developmentally challenged individuals, as well as individuals with auditory neuropathy, are special populations that may require more innovative approaches to aural rehabilitation. The future of implantable auditory devices is bright. This issue of *Otolaryngologic Clinics of North America* provides details on what is currently available as well as a glimpse into what is to come in the relatively near future. As at least some of these devices are not fully covered by health insurance in the United States, it is important for the counseling physician to understand the pertinent financial considerations and what is needed to promote accessibility.

Otolaryngol Clin N Am 52 (2019) xv–xvi
https://doi.org/10.1016/j.otc.2018.11.018
0030-6665/19/© 2019 Elsevier Inc. All rights reserved.

As the Guest Editors of this issue, Dr Chandrasekhar and I want our readers to be comfortable in considering all hearing rehabilitation options available. That task can be onerous, and we hope that the concise but complete treatment of the topics in this *Otolaryngologic Clinics of North America* issue streamlines the process. Important points to keep in mind while reading these articles are as follows:

1. Indications between devices greatly overlap.
2. Each company promotes their product as the best and safest; it is up to the otolaryngology-audiology team to determine the safety, reliability, and auditory benefit experienced in their setting.
3. Physicians and audiologists should guide the patient based on individual medical and auditory status.
4. Other medical considerations (skin eczema, need for MRI scanning, and so forth), anatomy (skin/skull thickness), and patient lifestyle and location all play important roles in the decision-making process.
5. The surgical/audiology team needs to have the skillset not only to offer but also to provide ongoing care for the devices.
6. Nonmedical and nonaudiologic factors of importance include financial factors, including insurance coverage and the local and ongoing support of the company.

We are practicing Otolaryngology in an exciting time, when the options for hearing improvement are extensive, and where the quality-of-life outcomes from these options are excellent. We all strive to stay on top of the latest advancements in our field. It is our hope that this issue of *Otolaryngologic Clinics of North America* on Implantable Hearing Devices helps you and your hearing health care team do just that.

Darius Kohan, MD
Lenox Hill Hospital/
Manhattan Eye Ear Nose Throat Hospital -Northwell Health System
NYU School of Medicine
863 Park Avenue
Suite 1East
New York, NY 10016, USA

Sujana S. Chandrasekhar, MD
ENT and Allergy Associates, LLP
18 East 48th Street, 2nd Floor
New York, NY 10017, USA

E-mail addresses:
earmaven@aol.com (D. Kohan)
ssc@nyotology.com (S.S. Chandrasekhar)

Medical and Audiological Indications for Implantable Auditory Devices

Maja Svrakic, MD, MSEd*, Andrea Vambutas, MD

KEYWORDS

- Implantable auditory device • Active acoustic implant • Active middle ear implant
- Direct acoustic stimulator • Bone-conducting device
- Active acoustic implant indications • Vibroplasty

KEY POINTS

- Active acoustic implants include bone-conducting devices, active middle ear implants, and direct acoustic cochlear stimulators.
- Medical indications for implantable devices can include hearing loss of various congenital, acquired, infectious, inflammatory, metabolic, neoplastic, traumatic, and iatrogenic etiologies.
- Audiological indications for implantable auditory devices are conductive, mixed, or sensorineural hearing loss that is mild to severe in degree.
- Currently, the indications for active middle ear implants (AMEIs) are mainly related to intolerance of conventional hearing aids, such as from chronic otitis externa or patient preference, severe mixed hearing losses with a destructed middle ear, failed revision surgeries in chronic otitis media, and congenital atresia.
- Rehabilitation with any of the surgically implanted devices must consider the etiology, type and severity of hearing loss, patient expectations and preferences, and a careful consideration of alternative and more traditional options.

INTRODUCTION

Implantable auditory devices (IADs) are active implants different from passive ones, such as ossicular chain prostheses. Active acoustic implants transduce acoustic sound energy to the cochlear perilymph either through skull vibration, via the ossicular chain, or by direct stimulation of the perilymph. Cochlear implants (CIs) and auditory brainstem implants (ABIs), in contrast, stimulate the cochlear nerve or brainstem

Disclosure Statement: The authors have no relevant financial disclosures.
Department of Otolaryngology, Long Island Jewish Medical Center, Hearing and Speech Center, Northwell Health, 430 Lakeville Road, New Hyde Park, NY 11042, USA
* Corresponding author.
E-mail address: msvrakic@northwell.edu

nuclei electrically. This article primarily considers the medical and audiological indications for active acoustic implants, including bone-conducting devices (BCDs), active middle ear implants (AMEIs), and direct acoustic cochlear stimulators (DACSs).

Devices and Definitions

Not all devices described here are commercially available or approved for implantation in the United States by the US Food and Drug Administration (FDA) but are approved in the European Union with a CE mark. They are all included to provide the broadest selection of auditory rehabilitation options available. **Table 1** summarizes the devices that will be discussed.

MEDICAL INDICATIONS
Ear Canal

Acquired stenosis
Soft tissue stenosis of the external auditory canal can occur from a variety of causes: infection, inflammation, trauma, and radiation. Bony stenosis is seen with exostoses and osteomas (**Fig. 1**). The stenosis, when complete, can cause a significant (>30 dB) conductive loss. Standard surgical treatment of soft tissue stenosis, even in experienced hands, results in restenosis in 10% to 20% of cases.[1]

Passive, active, percutaneous, or transcutaneous BCD can be offered, either as primary management strategy or if restenosis occurs.[2,3] Choice of device relies on the status of the patient's skin and quality of bone. AMEIs or DACSs have not been used in auditory rehabilitation of acquired stenosis of the ear canal.

Congenital aural atresia
Nonsyndromic congenital atresia of the ear canal most commonly occurs in the setting of a normal inner ear (**Fig. 2**) and preserved sensorineural hearing function, with few exceptions.[4] In lieu of atresiaplasty, the less extensive surgical BCD is an option for all patients desiring auditory rehabilitation.[3,5] BCDs are implanted after the age of 5, as the growing cranium typically reaches the necessary thickness at this time. Prior to age 5, BCDs can be used with a Softband as a nonsurgical alternative for hearing, speech, and language development, until surgery.

Selection of CAA patients who would benefit from atresiaplasty, and ossicular reconstruction or mobilization surgery involves use of established grading systems, looking at success of the ossiculoplasty with a passive prosthesis, and weighing the risks of injury (sensorineural hearing loss, facial nerve palsy) and restenosis.[6]

The role of AMEIs in auditory rehabilitation of atresia has only recently been explored.[7–15] Either fully[14,15] or partially[9,10,14] implantable devices have been placed on the incus, stapes, or the round window. When considering AMEI in CAA, special attention is given to the location of the facial nerve at the oval window, the inferior displacement of the tegmen mastoideum, pneumatization, and size of the middle ear space and the size of the surgical "corridors" to the stapes, oval window and round window.[16] The auditory advantage of rehabilitation with an AMEI over a BCD is still under investigation, although both types of devices carry more reliable results than does atresiaplasty surgery.[5,7,8,11]

Surgically closed ear canal
Any of the BCDs can be used in patients after temporal bone resection or closure of the ear canal (**Fig. 3**).[17–20] For patients who will also need radiation therapy, timing of the BCD placement should be considered, as radiation-related changes can compromise osseointegration and impede wound healing.[21]

Table 1
Features, common indications, and disadvantages of active acoustic implants

Type	Features	Examples	Common Indications	Disadvantages
Bone Conduction Devices (BCDs)				

Skin-drive	• Short, superficial surgery
	• External processor with internal magnet secured to mastoid bone
	• Osseointegration
	  ○ FDA: 3 mo
	  ○ Practice: 3–4 wk
	• >5 y of age (FDA)
		Baha Attract (Cochlear)
		Sophono (Medtronic)
			• SSD
			• Mild-moderate conductive and mixed hearing loss
			• Chronic ear disease
			• Actively draining/infected ears
			• Congenital atresia
			• Ear canal stenosis
				• MRI incompatibility
				• Transcutaneous energy loss

Direct-drive	• Short, superficial surgery • External processor on exteriorized (percutaneous) abutment secured to mastoid bone • Osseointegration – same as above • >5 y of age (FDA) • MRI compatible	Baha Connect (Cochlear) Ponto (Oticon)	• Same as skin-drive • Radiated bone	• Abutment always visible • Possible skin infections, overgrowth
Direct-drive Active	• External processor magnetically attaches to internal transducer secured to mastoid bone • Lower pressure on skin • Improved compliance • >5 y of age (EU CE mark) • >18 y of age (FDA)	Bonebridge (MedEl)	• Same as skin-drive	• MRI incompatibility • Requires favorable mastoid anatomy • Preoperative planning with CT scan needed
Light Activated Hearing Devices				
Laser photoemitter	• Short in-office procedure • Microphone, processor and emitter worn like a traditional hearing aid • Photodetector and actuator placed on ear drum • Easily removable • >18 y of age (FDA)	Earlen (Earlens Corporation)	• Moderate-severe sensorineural hearing loss • Inadequate gain or feedback with traditional hearing aid	• Contraindicated in chronic/active otitis media or otitis externa or TM perforation

(continued on next page)

Table 1
(continued)

Type	Features	Examples	Common Indications	Disadvantages
Active Middle Ear Implants				

Partially implantable External processor	• External processor with internal floating mass transducer
	• Internal component can couple to ossicular chain, round window, oval window
	• Soundbridge:
	  >5 y (EU CE mark)
	  >18 y (FDA)
	• MET
	  >14 y (EU CE mark)
		Vibrant Soundbridge (MedEl)
		MET (Cochlear)
		Not FDA approved
			• Moderate-severe to severe conductive or mixed hearing loss
			• Chronic ear disease with poor auditory outcomes after ossiculoplasty
			• Congenital atresia
			• Advanced otosclerosis
				• MRI incompatibility
				• Contraindicated in active middle ear disease, tumors, radiation
				• Longer, more technical surgery
				• Adequate mastoid and ME space required

Partially implantable In the canal processor	• In the canal processor with floating mass transducer • Straightforward, transcanal procedure • >18 y (FDA)	Maxum (Ototronix)	• Moderate-to-severe sensorineural hearing loss • Intact ossicular chain, mobile stapes	• MRI incompatibility • Contraindicated in stapes fixation in addition to contraindications listed previously
Fully implantable	• Internal sensor and transducer couple to ossicular chain • Internal processor secured to mastoid temporal bone • Carina: >14 y (EU CE mark) • Envoy: >18 y (FDA)	Carina (Cochlear) Not FDA approved Envoy (Esteem)	• Moderate-severe to severe sensorineural, mixed or conductive hearing loss • Patients desiring cosmesis and convenience, poor tolerance of hearing aid	• MRI incompatibility • Contraindicated in active middle ear disease, tumors, radiation • Long, technically challenging mastoid and middle ear surgery • Limited battery life; requires reoperation for battery change • Contraindicated in osteodegenerative disorders
Direct Acoustic Cochlear Stimulator				
Partially implantable	• External processor with internal actuator/transducer placed on oval, round or a 3rd window • >18 y of age (EU CE mark)	Codacs (Cochlear) Not FDA approved	• Severe-to-profound mixed hearing loss • Advanced obliterative otosclerosis • Chronic ear disease with poor auditory outcomes after ossiculoplasty	• Contraindicated in active middle ear disease, tumors, radiation • Longer, more technical surgery • Adequate ME and mastoid space required

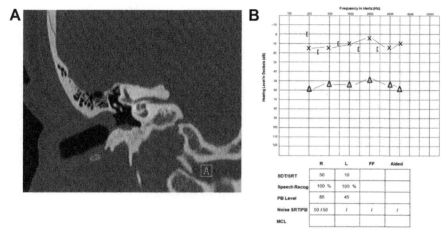

Fig. 1. Acquired ear canal stenosis. 52-year-old woman with right complete fibrous stenosis of the ear canal as a result of chronic otitis externa. Coronal computed tomography (CT) scan of the temporal bone (A) demonstrates the soft tissue stenosis. A pure tone audiogram with thresholds and word recognition scores (B) shows a moderate-severe conductive hearing loss.

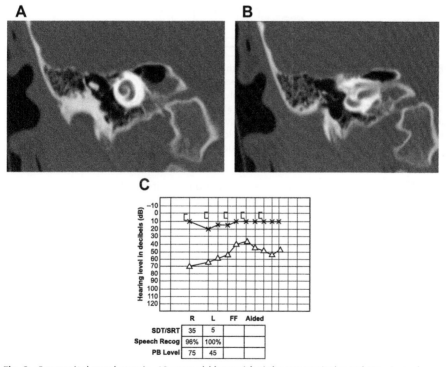

Fig. 2. Congenital aural atresia. 12-year-old boy with right congenital aural atresia and normally formed auricle. Sequential coronal sequences of a CT scan (A, B) demonstrate complete bony atresia with otherwise favorable anatomy and no cochlear abnormalities. The audiogram (C) shows a moderate to moderate-severe conductive hearing loss.

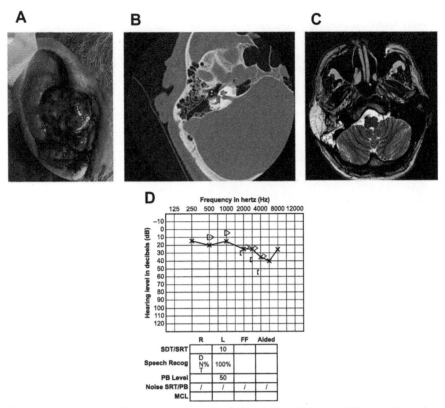

Fig. 3. Auricular cancer. 55-year-old man with right spindle cell cancer of the auricle and ear canal. The intraoperative photograph shows a large exophytic mass (*A*). The underlying temporal bone is well aerated without involvement of the middle ear or mastoid (*B*). Postoperative MRI (*C*) demonstrates a complete auriculectomy, lateral temporal bone resection, and obliteration of the ear canal. Preoperative audiogram (*D*) shows a likely mixed hearing loss with near maximal conductive hearing loss; air thresholds could not be performed on the right ear because of the patient's obstructing lesion.

AMEIs have been successfully used after subtotal petrosectomies with obliterated ear canals by placement of the FMT on the round window[18,22,23] or the stapes head,[24] either at primary surgery or subsequently. Their durability in radiated temporal bones is not known. In cases where disease needs MRI surveillance, MRI-compatible BCDs are the implants of choice.

Tympanic Membrane

Perforation

Owing to the excellent results of type 1 tympanoplasty, most patients would not choose auditory devices for perforation-related conductive hearing loss (CHL). Further, AMEIs and DACSs are contraindicated in tympanic membrane (TM) perforations, active middle ear disease, or external otitis.[25] Tympanoplasty with or without ossiculoplasty should be performed first. If the hearing is not satisfactory, and the patient's ear is free of infections, an AMEI can be placed on whichever part of the ossicular chain is intact, or at the round window. Alternatively, BCDs can be used, either with or without the repair of the eardrum, and can be performed as a single surgery.

Ossicular Chain

Chronic otitis media

The priority in treating chronic ear disease is creating a safe, dry ear. Once this is accomplished, audiologic rehabilitation becomes the next goal. Results of ossiculoplasty in cases of chronic ear disease are varied, and at best over 40% of patients will have greater than 20 dB of ABG,[26,27] independent of the reconstructive technique.[28] In these cases, active devices have superior outcomes.[29]

Successful use of BCDs in chronic otitis media (COM) has been well established.[3,30,31] Vibroplasty, the middle ear reconstructive surgery performed with active acoustic implants such as AMEIs, shows promise in chronic ear disease, especially in patients with mixed hearing losses. Coupling to a discontinuous or reconstructed ossicular chain,[32–34] or the round window[35,36] is possible.[37] In COM, the anatomy may be constricted, and preoperative imaging will guide the surgeon if considering AMEI, particularly the fully implantable devices (**Fig. 4**).

Otosclerosis

The outcome of a standard stapes surgery for otosclerosis causing a predominantly conductive hearing loss is predictably good.[38] For active implantable devices to be appealing, they should either be fully implantable or be able to address associated sensorineural hearing loss (SNHL). BCDs, therefore, are not a common choice in these patients, although they have been used for this indication.[31,39]

The fully implantable cochlear Carina requires longer operating time, is more technically difficult, and is associated with more complications than the standard stapes surgery with a passive implant. However, in cases of multiple revision surgeries and poor accessibility because of scarring, round window placement of a Carina-type device has been successful.[40]

Vibroplasty of the long process of the incus[41] or the round window[42–45] has been successful in treating mixed hearing loss caused by otosclerosis, specifically in patients who could not tolerate the occlusion effect of the hearing aid, had concurrent chronic ear disease or poor auditory outcomes with the hearing aid.

For advanced otosclerosis with SNHL (**Fig. 5**), the patient has an option of combining the standard stapes surgery with a traditional hearing aid versus a cochlear

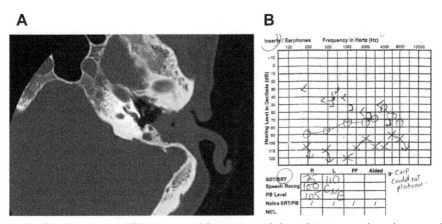

Fig. 4. Chronic otomastoiditis. 61-year-old woman with branchio-oto-renal syndrome and bilateral mixed hearing loss. Left ear is status after tympanomastoidectomy with ossicular chain reconstruction (*A*) and poor audiological result (*B*).

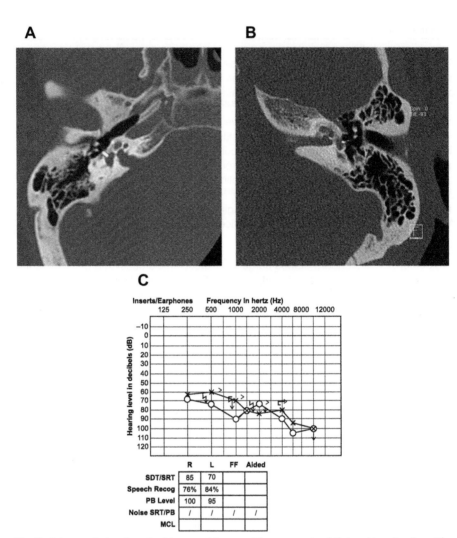

Fig. 5. Advanced otosclerosis. 64-year-old man with progressive bilateral hearing loss. The axial CT images demonstrate stapes prostheses bilaterally as well as signs of advanced otospongiosis involving the otic capsule (*A, B*). His audiogram (*C*) shows severe sensorineural hearing loss with good speech recognition scores and a surgically closed air bone gap.

implant, and, more recently a DACS device.[46,47] DACS has shown superiority over traditional hearing aids in cases of moderate-to-severe mixed hearing loss in otosclerosis.[48] DACS can also be used to stimulate the cochlea via a third window, especially in cases of round and oval window obliteration, although this has been shown on an animal model only.[49]

For a related but molecularly distinct pathology of osteogenesis imperfecta, results with a standard stapes surgery have been disappointing, mostly because of the progression of SNHL.[50] Osteogenesis imperfecta has been successfully treated with a stapes vibroplasty in 2 cases,[51] with the added advantage of addressing the SNHL.

Congenital ossicular fixation

For the relatively rare cases of congenitally fixed stapes or juvenile otosclerosis, standard stapes surgery is less successful than for adult otosclerosis, with a closure of the ABG to within 10 dB occurring in only 50% to 60% of cases.[52] Stapes surgery is significantly more successful (>80%) in cases of isolated juvenile otosclerosis versus in those with a congenitally fixed stapes, especially when associated with other ossicular malformations.[52,53] For mallear or incudal fixation without associated stapes anomalies, passive implants are successful in closing the ABG in greater than 90% of cases.[54]

Vibroplasty for congenitally fixed ossicular chain that is not caused by aural atresia has not been studied. However, there may be a role for AMEIs in patients who either fail ossiculoplasty or have a higher likelihood of poor results, cannot tolerate hearing aids, or have mixed hearing loss (MHL).

Traumatic ossicular dislocation

Ossicular chain trauma with primarily CHL can be rehabilitated well with a standard ossiculoplasty.[55] However, in cases of traumatic MHL, seen with stapedial dislocation or footplate fracture (**Fig. 6**), the results are more variable.[54,55]

These patients have a choice of tympanoplasty with a hearing aid or a BCD, AMEI, DACS, or CI, depending on the severity of SNHL. There are no data on AMEI or DACS for this indication.

Middle ear tumors

In cases of middle ear tumors, important considerations are the likelihood of disease recurrence or progression, need for any adjuvant treatments such as radiation therapy, size of the tumor and structures involved, pre-existing or resultant SNHL, and need for surveillance with MRI. With paragangliomas (**Fig. 7**), for example, good audiological results have been achieved after tumor removal and with ossicular chain reconstruction.[56,57] For rarer tumors, such as adenomatous tumors of the middle ear, similar rehabilitation principles are applied.[58]

As most active implants are not MRI-compatible, and hearing outcomes are generally good with traditional ossicular reconstruction, early implantation of these types of devices is probably not indicated. Once the hearing result has stabilized and tumor recurrence ruled out, and if the patient either has a persistent auditory deficit, cannot tolerate a hearing aid, or has MHL, BCD, AMEI, DACS, or CI type devices could

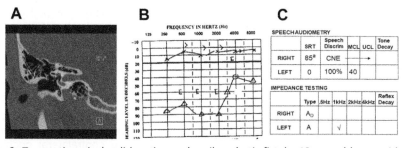

Fig. 6. Traumatic ossicular dislocation and perilymphatic fistula. 18-year-old man with right hearing loss and dizziness after Q-tip induced trauma. Air in the vestibule indicates a likely stapes footplate fracture, which was discovered intraoperatively (*A*). The perilymph leak resulted in a mixed hearing loss on the right side (*B*), decreased speech discrimination score, and an A_D type tympanometry caused by ossicular dislocation (*C*). [a] masked pt could not tolerate sound.

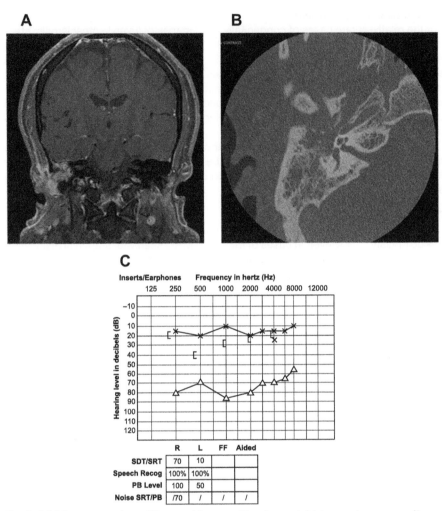

Fig. 7. Middle ear neoplasm. 34-year-old man with a large right tympanic paraganglioma, showing enhancement on the coronal MRI (*A*), tracking along the temporal bone and the facial nerve. CT scan (*B*) demonstrates the associated bony destruction. The patient presented with right facial nerve paralysis and ipsilateral conductive hearing loss (*C*).

theoretically be used depending on the degree and type of hearing loss and patient preference.

Inner Ear

Implantable auditory devices may be used in instances of unilateral sensorineural hearing loss (ie, single-sided deafness [SSD]), where the contralateral cochlea has normal, or near-normal hearing. In these cases, a BCD transmits information to the contralateral cochlea. Surgical discussions regarding these devices should be balanced, as these devices do not stimulate the ipsilateral cochlea, and function similar to CROS (contralateral routing of sound) or BiCROS (bidirectional contralateral routing of sound) hearing aid technology. In 1 study of 196 patients with single-sided sensorineural deafness, 66% of these patients declined a bone-anchored hearing device after the trial period; the predominant reason was lack of improvement of understanding speech in noise.[59] These devices can provide substantial benefit to some patients who cannot benefit from conventional hearing aids because of poor or absent speech discrimination scores in the ipsilateral ear. A test trial of the device can be done in the office, audiology booth, and even out in a noisy environment, to ensure adequate presurgical expectations. Patient satisfaction with BCDs for SSD is substantially poorer than satisfaction with BCDs for conductive pathology.[60]

In conditions of bilateral SNHL, AMEIs or LAHDs may be used to stimulate the ipsilateral cochlea for those patients with stable sensorineural hearing loss who do not meet criteria for cochlear implantation. Cochlear implants are now used freely in Europe and in selected cases in the United States for SSD and can provide true binaurality. Implantable auditory devices discussed here would continue to be of benefit in patients with SSD as a result of cochlear nerve pathology.

Inner ear malformations
Inner ear malformations may include enlarged vestibular aqueduct, Mondini malformations, common cavity deformities (within the Mondini spectrum), cochlear aplasia/hypoplasia, and narrow internal auditory canals. When unilateral pathology exists, and the contralateral ear is normal, implantable auditory devices can provide substantial benefit, and direct drive and transcutaneous BCD devices have remained the most commonly used IADs. Caution is advised when considering non-CI IADs in patients with bilateral inner ear malformations, as these etiologies are likely to cause progressive sensorineural loss.

Congenital sensorineural hearing loss
Most patients with congenital SNHL benefit from conventional hearing aids or Cis. They could use AMEI, but data are poor, as these devices are approved only after age 14 for this indication.

Presbycusis
Age-related SNHL, or presbycusis, usually presents as a high-frequency, symmetric SNHL. Similar to congenital SNHL, most patients with presbycusis benefit from conventional amplification. Partially or fully implantable AMEI systems may be used in presbycusis for aesthetic or lifestyle concerns, and for the auditory advantages discussed in later articles. These are excellent candidates, as their hearing loss is largely stable, and their ear anatomy is normal.

Meniere disease and immune-mediated hearing loss
In both Meniere disease and autoimmune inner ear disease (AIED), most patients present with an asymmetric possibly fluctuating sensorineural hearing loss. Because of the potentially unstable hearing loss, implantable auditory devices are to be used with caution in these patients. Other considerations are as previously mentioned for SNHL. In patients who feel debilitated by frequent and severe fluctuations in hearing loss, especially if associated with vertigo, a CI may be the best option even if contralateral hearing is normal.

Sudden sensorineural hearing loss
Patients who do not recover from sudden severe-profound SNHL may obtain benefit from either a BCD or CI for SSD, as discussed previously.

Auditory Nerve and Brainstem

BCDs provide good-to-excellent benefit for patients with cochlear nerve or brainstem hearing loss, no matter the cause, if there is adequate cochlear reserve in the contralateral ear. One study of BCD for SSD after vestibular schwannoma resection showed 17% improvement in background noise and 12% improvement in ease of communication.[61] As mentioned previously, these patients may meet expanded criteria for CI, which would offer ipsilateral hearing and not CROS-type benefit.

AUDIOLOGICAL INDICATIONS
Pure Tone Average Thresholds

The following diagram can be used to determine some of the options in rehabilitation of audiological function with respect to pure tone thresholds (**Fig. 8**). Purely conductive hearing losses (ABG >30 dB, dbSNHL <30 dB) lend themselves well to BCDs. Mixed hearing losses can be rehabilitated with BCD, AMEI, and DACS type devices, depending on the degree of total and sensorineural hearing loss. LAHDs and Maxum AMEIs have been used in patients with primary SNHL.[62,63] CIs are the best option for severe to profound SNHL.

Speech Discrimination Scores

For speech discrimination scores less than 40%, cochlear implants are the best choice. AMEIs and DACSs have been used in patients with preoperative speech scores in the 40% to 70% range, yielding an improvement in speech reception threshold of 40 dB.[64] AMEIs seem to provide greater improvements in speech recognition and quality of life[65] over hearing aids, particularly in these more difficult hearing situations.

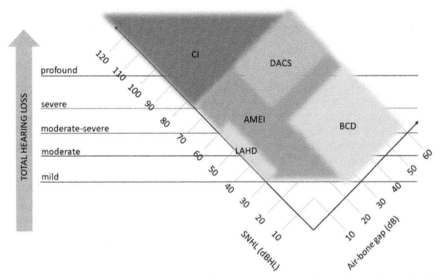

Fig. 8. Pure tone audiometry indications for active implants. dB, decibel; dBHL, decibel hearing loss; LAHD, light activated hearing device. (*Adapted from* Cochlear Limited. Advances in middle ear implants and direct acoustic cochlear implants. Sound Connection. 2016;11. Available at: https://www.cochlear.com/uk/for-professionals/sound-connection/advances-in-middle-ear-implants-and-direct-acoustic-cochlear-implants; with permission. Accessed December 14, 2018.)

Unilateral Hearing Loss

If there is a near normal hearing threshold on the contralateral ear, most patients do not report a high subjective benefit for AMEIs, which is why they are indicated for bilateral hearing losses. BCDs continue to be used for unilateral single-sided SNHL.

Stability of Hearing and Onset of Hearing Loss

AMEI or DACS devices should not be implanted in patients with unstable or fluctuating hearing loss; these patients benefit initially from adjustable traditional hearing aids. If the hearing loss deteriorates to severe loss, CIs have resulted in excellent outcomes. Patients with prelingual hearing loss are optimized with CI.

Patient Preference

As with all hearing technologies, patient preference and shared decision-making are paramount. Even though patients may prefer them for cosmesis and convenience, fully implantable devices have not shown audiological equivalence to conventional hearing aids.[66] A significant advantage to many, but not all, of the IADs, similar to conventional hearing aids, is the patient's ability to touch and feel and even test the device to some extent prior to committing to surgery.

SUMMARY

Current indications for AMEIs are mainly related to intolerance of conventional hearing aids, severe mixed hearing loss with abnormal middle ear anatomy, and certain conditions where traditional surgical reconstruction has inconsistent results.[12] Rehabilitation with any of the surgically implanted devices must take into account the etiology, type and severity of hearing loss, patient expectations and preferences, and a careful consideration of alternative and more traditional options.

REFERENCES

1. Luong A, Roland PS. Acquired external auditory canal stenosis: assessment and management. Curr Opin Otolaryngol Head Neck Surg 2005;13(5):273–6.
2. Lustig LR, Arts HA, Brackmann DE, et al. Hearing rehabilitation using the BAHA bone-anchored hearing aid: results in 40 patients. Otol Neurotol 2001;22(3):328–34.
3. Sprinzl GM, Wolf-Magele A. The Bonebridge bone conduction hearing implant: indication criteria, surgery and a systematic review of the literature. Clin Otolaryngol 2016;41(2):131–43.
4. Halle TR, Soares BP, Todd NW. Inner ear anomalies in children with isolated unilateral congenital aural atresia. Int J Pediatr Otorhinolaryngol 2017;95:5–8.
5. Farnoosh S, Mitsinikos FT, Maceri D, et al. Bone-anchored hearing aid vs. reconstruction of the external auditory canal in children and adolescents with congenital aural atresia: a comparison study of outcomes. Front Pediatr 2014;2:5.
6. Service GJ, Roberson JB Jr. Current concepts in repair of aural atresia. Curr Opin Otolaryngol Head Neck Surg 2010;18(6):536–8.
7. Agterberg MJ, Frenzel H, Wollenberg B, et al. Amplification options in unilateral aural atresia: an active middle ear implant or a bone conduction device? Otol Neurotol 2014;35(1):129–35.
8. Dazert S, Thomas JP, Volkenstein S. Surgical and technical modalities for hearing restoration in ear malformations. Facial Plast Surg 2015;31(6):581–6.
9. Frenzel H, Hanke F, Beltrame M, et al. Application of the Vibrant Soundbridge to unilateral osseous atresia cases. Laryngoscope 2009;119(1):67–74.

10. Kiefer J, Arnold W, Staudenmaier R. Round window stimulation with an implantable hearing aid (Soundbridge) combined with autogenous reconstruction of the auricle - a new approach. ORL J Otorhinolaryngol Relat Spec 2006;68(6): 378–85.

11. Lo JF, Tsang WS, Yu JY, et al. Contemporary hearing rehabilitation options in patients with aural atresia. Biomed Res Int 2014;2014:761579.

12. Luers JC, Huttenbrink KB. Vibrant Soundbridge rehabilitation of conductive and mixed hearing loss. Otolaryngol Clin North Am 2014;47(6):915–26.

13. Roman S, Denoyelle F, Farinetti A, et al. Middle ear implant in conductive and mixed congenital hearing loss in children. Int J Pediatr Otorhinolaryngol 2012; 76(12):1775–8.

14. Siegert R, Mattheis S, Kasic J. Fully implantable hearing aids in patients with congenital auricular atresia. Laryngoscope 2007;117(2):336–40.

15. Verhaert N, Fuchsmann C, Tringali S, et al. Strategies of active middle ear implants for hearing rehabilitation in congenital aural atresia. Otol Neurotol 2011; 32(4):639–45.

16. Frenzel H, Sprinzl G, Widmann G, et al. Grading system for the selection of patients with congenital aural atresia for active middle ear implants. Neuroradiology 2013;55(7):895–911.

17. Bibas AG, Gleeson MJ. Bilateral squamous cell carcinoma of the temporal bones. Skull Base 2006;16(4):213–8.

18. Linder T, Schlegel C, DeMin N, et al. Active middle ear implants in patients undergoing subtotal petrosectomy: new application for the Vibrant Soundbridge device and its implication for lateral cranium base surgery. Otol Neurotol 2009;30(1): 41–7.

19. Gluth MB, Friedman AB, Atcherson SR, et al. Hearing aid tolerance after revision and obliteration of canal wall down mastoidectomy cavities. Otol Neurotol 2013; 34(4):711–4.

20. Ketelslagers K, Somers T, De Foer B, et al. Results, hearing rehabilitation, and follow-up with magnetic resonance imaging after tympanomastoid exenteration, obliteration, and external canal overclosure for severe chronic otitis media. Ann Otol Rhinol Laryngol 2007;116(9):705–11.

21. Soo G, Tong MC, Tsang WS, et al. The BAHA hearing system for hearing-impaired postirradiated nasopharyngeal cancer patients: a new indication. Otol Neurotol 2009;30(4):496–501.

22. Henseler MA, Polanski JF, Schlegel C, et al. Active middle ear implants in patients undergoing subtotal petrosectomy: long-term follow-up. Otol Neurotol 2014; 35(3):437–41.

23. Verhaert N, Mojallal H, Schwab B. Indications and outcome of subtotal petrosectomy for active middle ear implants. Eur Arch Otorhinolaryngol 2013;270(4): 1243–8.

24. Liu Q, Feng G, Shang Y, et al. Vibrant Soundbridge implantation: floating mass transducer coupled with the stapes head and embedded in fat. ORL J Otorhinolaryngol Relat Spec 2018;80(2):159–64.

25. Zwartenkot JW, Mulder JJ, Snik AF, et al. Vibrant Soundbridge surgery in patients with severe external otitis: complications of a transcanal approach. Otol Neurotol 2011;32(3):398–402.

26. Nevoux J, Roger G, Chauvin P, et al. Cartilage shield tympanoplasty in children: review of 268 consecutive cases. Arch Otolaryngol Head Neck Surg 2011;137(1): 24–9.

27. O'Connell BP, Rizk HG, Hutchinson T, et al. Long-term outcomes of titanium ossi-culoplasty in chronic otitis media. Otolaryngol Head Neck Surg 2016;154(6): 1084–92.

28. Demir UL, Karaca S, Ozmen OA, et al. Is it the middle ear disease or the recon-struction material that determines the functional outcome in ossicular chain reconstruction? Otol Neurotol 2012;33(4):580–5.

29. Lee JM, Jung J, Moon IS, et al. Benefits of active middle ear implants in mixed hearing loss: stapes versus round window. Laryngoscope 2017;127(6):1435–41.

30. Macnamara M, Phillips D, Proops DW. The bone anchored hearing aid (BAHA) in chronic suppurative otitis media (CSOM). J Laryngol Otol Suppl 1996;21:38–40.

31. McLarnon CM, Davison T, Johnson IJ. Bone-anchored hearing aid: comparison of benefit by patient subgroups. Laryngoscope 2004;114(5):942–4.

32. Gostian AO, Huttenbrink KB, Luers JC, et al. Long-term results of TORP-vibro-plasty. Otol Neurotol 2015;36(6):1054–60.

33. Huttenbrink KB, Beutner D, Bornitz M, et al. Clip vibroplasty: experimental eval-uation and first clinical results. Otol Neurotol 2011;32(4):650–3.

34. Huttenbrink KB, Beutner D, Zahnert T. Clinical results with an active middle ear implant in the oval window. Adv Otorhinolaryngol 2010;69:27–31.

35. Edfeldt L, Stromback K, Grendin J, et al. Evaluation of cost-utility in middle ear implantation in the 'Nordic School': a multicenter study in Sweden and Norway. Acta Otolaryngol 2014;134(1):19–25.

36. Rajan GP, Lampacher P, Ambett R, et al. Impact of floating mass transducer coupling and positioning in round window vibroplasty. Otol Neurotol 2011; 32(2):271–7.

37. Beleites T, Neudert M, Bornitz M, et al. Sound transfer of active middle ear im-plants. Otolaryngol Clin North Am 2014;47(6):859–91.

38. Sevy A, Arriaga M. The stapes prosthesis: past, present, and future. Otolaryngol Clin North Am 2018;51(2):393–404.

39. Bianchin G, Bonali M, Russo M, et al. Active bone conduction system: outcomes with the Bonebridge transcutaneous device. ORL J Otorhinolaryngol Relat Spec 2015;77(1):17–26.

40. Martin C, Deveze A, Richard C, et al. European results with totally implantable ca-rina placed on the round window: 2-year follow-up. Otol Neurotol 2009;30(8): 1196–203.

41. Gregoire A, Van Damme JP, Gilain C, et al. Our auditory results using the Vibrant Soundbridge on the long process of the incus: 20 years of data. Auris Nasus Lar-ynx 2018;45(1):66–72.

42. Beltrame AM, Martini A, Prosser S, et al. Coupling the Vibrant Soundbridge to co-chlea round window: auditory results in patients with mixed hearing loss. Otol Neurotol 2009;30(2):194–201.

43. Coordes A, Jahreiss L, Schonfeld U, et al. Active middle ear implant coupled bilaterally to the round window despite bilateral implanted stapes prostheses. Laryngoscope 2017;127(2):500–3.

44. Venail F, Lavieille JP, Meller R, et al. New perspectives for middle ear implants: first results in otosclerosis with mixed hearing loss. Laryngoscope 2007;117(3):552–5.

45. Dumon T. Vibrant soundbridge middle ear implant in otosclerosis: technique - indication. Adv Otorhinolaryngol 2007;65:320–2.

46. Eshraghi AA, Ila K, Ocak E, et al. Advanced otosclerosis: stapes surgery or cochlear implantation? Otolaryngol Clin North Am 2018;51(2):429–40.

47. Hausler R, Stieger C, Bernhard H, et al. A novel implantable hearing system with direct acoustic cochlear stimulation. Audiol Neurootol 2008;13(4):247–56.

48. Busch S, Kruck S, Spickers D, et al. First clinical experiences with a direct acoustic cochlear stimulator in comparison to preoperative fitted conventional hearing aids. Otol Neurotol 2013;34(9):1711–8.
49. Lupo JE, Koka K, Jenkins HA, et al. Third-window vibroplasty with an active middle ear implant: assessment of physiologic responses in a model of stapes fixation in Chinchilla lanigera. Otol Neurotol 2012;33(3):425–31.
50. Garretsen TJ, Cremers CW. Stapes surgery in osteogenesis imperfecta: analysis of postoperative hearing loss. Ann Otol Rhinol Laryngol 1991;100(2):120–30.
51. Kontorinis G, Lenarz T, Mojallal H, et al. Power stapes: an alternative method for treating hearing loss in osteogenesis imperfecta? Otol Neurotol 2011;32(4): 589–95.
52. Asik B, Binar M, Serdar M, et al. A meta-analysis of surgical success rates in congenital stapes fixation and juvenile otosclerosis. Laryngoscope 2016;126(1): 191–8.
53. Carlson ML, Van Abel KM, Pelosi S, et al. Outcomes comparing primary pediatric stapedectomy for congenital stapes footplate fixation and juvenile otosclerosis. Otol Neurotol 2013;34(5):816–20.
54. Park GY, Choi JE, Cho YS. Traumatic ossicular disruption with isolated fracture of the stapes suprastructure: comparison with incudostapedial joint dislocation. Acta Otolaryngol 2014;134(12):1225–30.
55. Delrue S, Verhaert N, Dinther JV, et al. Surgical management and hearing outcome of traumatic ossicular injuries. J Int Adv Otol 2016;12(3):231–6.
56. Medina M, Prasad SC, Patnaik U, et al. The effects of tympanomastoid paragangliomas on hearing and the audiological outcomes after surgery over a long-term follow-up. Audiol Neurootol 2014;19(5):342–50.
57. Papaspyrou K, Mewes T, Toth M, et al. Hearing results after hypotympanotomy for glomus tympanicum tumors. Otol Neurotol 2011;32(2):291–6.
58. Pelosi S, Koss S. Adenomatous tumors of the middle ear. Otolaryngol Clin North Am 2015;48(2):305–15.
59. Baguley DM, Bird J, Humphriss RL, et al. The evidence base for the application of contralateral bone anchored hearing aids in acquired unilateral sensorineural hearing loss in adults. Clin Otolaryngol 2006;31(1):6–14.
60. Tringali S, Grayeli AB, Bouccara D, et al. A survey of satisfaction and use among patients fitted with a BAHA. Eur Arch Otorhinolaryngol 2008;265(12):1461–4.
61. House JW, Kutz JW Jr, Chung J, et al. Bone-anchored hearing aid subjective benefit for unilateral deafness. Laryngoscope 2010;120(3):601–7.
62. Fay JP, Perkins R, Levy SC, et al. Preliminary evaluation of a light-based contact hearing device for the hearing impaired. Otol Neurotol 2013;34(5):912–21.
63. Gantz BJ, Perkins R, Murray M, et al. Light-driven contact hearing aid for broad-spectrum amplification: safety and effectiveness pivotal study. Otol Neurotol 2017;38(3):352–9.
64. Lenarz T, Zwartenkot JW, Stieger C, et al. Multicenter study with a direct acoustic cochlear implant. Otol Neurotol 2013;34(7):1215–25.
65. Klein K, Nardelli A, Stafinski T. A systematic review of the safety and effectiveness of fully implantable middle ear hearing devices: the carina and esteem systems. Otol Neurotol 2012;33(6):916–21.
66. Savas VA, Gunduz B, Karamert R, et al. Comparison of Carina active middle-ear implant with conventional hearing aids for mixed hearing loss. J Laryngol Otol 2016;130(4):340–3.

Limitations of Conventional Hearing Aids

Examining Common Complaints and Issues that Can and Cannot Be Remedied

Sara Lerner, AuD*

KEYWORDS

- Hearing aids • Bone osseointegrated implants • Middle ear implants
- Acoustic feedback • Occlusion effect • Discomfort

KEY POINTS

- With modern hearing aids, clinicians can often reduce common hearing aid complaints, such as acoustic feedback and the occlusion effect and discomfort, without the need to recommend implantable devices.
- Reducing or eliminating the occlusion effect can make a hearing aid more susceptible to acoustic feedback and reducing acoustic feedback, in turn, may cause the occlusion effect.
- For patients with severe hearing loss or other unique circumstances that make conventional hearing aids difficult or uncomfortable to use, turning to middle ear implants or osseointegrated implants can be appropriate.

Conventional hearing aids (CHAs) undergo constant improvement and technological and cosmetic modification, and work well for most patients with hearing loss. However, there are a number of reasons CHAs may not work well for a particular patient and why implantable devices may be preferable for them. A patient's dissatisfaction with CHAs may be due to inadequate sound and/or speech amplification, visibility/cosmesis, and/or the inability to consistently wear the CHA owing to chronic otitis externa or middle ear disease. As an alternative to CHAs, osseointegrated implants (OI), initially approved by the US Food and Drug Administration in 1996 and subsequently expanded as approved for single-sided deafness (SSD),[1] or middle ear implants (MEIs), approved by the US Food and Drug Administration in 2001, help patients with conductive, mixed, or sensorineural hearing loss who have tried CHAs

Disclosure Statement: The author has nothing to disclose.
ENT and Allergy Associates, 261 5th Avenue, Suite 901, New York, NY 10016, USA
* 259 Grand Street, Apartment C, Jersey City, NJ 07302.
E-mail address: slerner@entandallergy.com

Otolaryngol Clin N Am 52 (2019) 211–220
https://doi.org/10.1016/j.otc.2018.11.002
0030-6665/19/© 2018 Elsevier Inc. All rights reserved.

with limited success or with dissatisfaction.[2] Some benefits of MEIs or OIs over CHAs are undeniable, such as the ability to be worn 24 hours per day (whereas CHAs must be removed for sleep), near or complete invisibility, and efficacy in atretic or other malformed ears. Additionally, OIs and MEIs are also often cited as superior to CHAs for their ability to eliminate feedback and the consequences of occlusion, and for solving the problem of a patient who frequently suffers from CHA-related ear infections or otherwise finds their CHA too uncomfortable to wear consistently.[1] This article explores what can be done clinically for CHA users suffering from excessive feedback, the occlusion effect, frequent ear infections, or CHA discomfort to optimize their use of CHA, and in what circumstances implantable devices are be a superior option.

The increased use of implantable devices in recent years suggests that, at least in some cases, CHA users are dissatisfied. MEIs are expensive relative to CHAs and even though OIs may be more affordable, because they are often covered through insurance, both types of implantable devices include an invasive procedure. Significant advances in CHA technology have, however, increased patient satisfaction, making the traditional complaints about CHA less common. MarkeTrak 9, a 2015 survey, found that overall CHA satisfaction increased from 74% in 2008 to 81% in 2015. Patient satisfaction was even higher for CHAs purchased in the last year at 91%. In 2015, more than one-half of repeat CHA buyers (51%) considered their CHAs to be much better than their previous CHAs, and 34% considered them somewhat better.[3] Technological advances since 2015 in CHAs, including improvements in signal processing and new features (eg, Bluetooth and automatic programs), have likely only increased satisfaction levels.

Complaints of feedback and the occlusion effect, which used to be prevalent, can now be addressed for the majority of CHA users without the need for an implantable device. The advances made in signal processing, when paired with expert fitting and dispensing of CHAs, can eliminate the effects of feedback and occlusion for most patients. Other complaints (eg, infections and general discomfort) and restraints (eg, gain requirements) can also be addressed successfully for many CHA users because there are many types, styles, and materials available for use in CHAs. This article examines and evaluates the methods, from an audiologist's perspective, of reducing these common complaints in patients with a CHA. These methods are often able to significantly reduce or eliminate feedback, occlusion effect, and discomfort and provide sufficient gain. However, for some patients remedying these issues may not be possible because they come with tradeoffs that make implantable devices more desirable options for specific patients.

OCCLUSION EFFECT

CHA users may have complaints about the sound of their own voice. They may find that their voice sounds hollow or "boomy," and it may sound like they are in a barrel. These complaints, in addition to complaints of other self-produced sounds having a similarly unpleasant reverberation or echo (eg, chewing), are due to the occlusion effect. The occlusion effect occurs when self-produced sounds are transmitted simultaneously via air conduction and bone conduction. When the ear canal is open, as is the case for individuals without CHAs, the increased sound pressure leaks out. However, when a CHA or ear mold blocks the ear canal, the increased sound pressure is retained in the ear canal, causing the occlusion effect.[4]

The degree of low-frequency hearing loss often determines whether or not an individual struggles with the occlusion effect. Individuals with a 60 decibels hearing level hearing loss in the low frequencies should not be bothered by the occlusion effect.

Because these individuals require significant low-frequency gain from the CHA, the increased sound of their own voice from the occlusion effect is not noticeable or unpleasant when coupled with the amplification already being provided by the CHA. The occlusion effect, however, is particularly troublesome to those with less than a 50 decibels hearing level low-frequency hearing loss.[5]

Ineffective, But Often Used, Methods for Reducing the Occlusion Effect

There are 2 common, yet ineffective, methods used to manage the occlusion effect that may propagate, rather than alleviate, complaints: (1) the "get used to it" approach and (2) lowering the low-frequency gain. A patient suffering from the occlusion effect is often counseled to get used to the new sound of their own voice. When the sound of their own voice is altered by the occlusion effect, acclimating to the "boomy" or hollow quality is nearly impossible, because the occlusion effect may increase the level of low-frequency sounds, such as vowels, upward of 20 to 30 dB.[5] Asking a patient to acclimate to this level of change is unreasonable and could lead to reduced CHA use. The other flawed method in reducing the occlusion effect is to lower the low-frequency gain. Some CHA manufacturers even have an "occlusion manager" feature in their software designed specifically for this purpose. The increased low-frequency sound from the occlusion effect does not come from the low-frequency gain from the CHA; rather, it is created from the closed off ear canal. Decreasing low-frequency gain will not decrease complaints of the occlusion effect, but only increase complaints of CHA ineffectiveness.[6]

Effective Methods for Minimizing or Eliminating the Occlusion Effect

There are, however, 2 methods that a clinician can use to eliminate the occlusion effect in patients: (1) venting and (2) deep insertion. In addition, if those methods are not feasible for the reasons detailed elsewhere in this article, a clinician can also try to increase low-frequency gain to decrease (but not eliminate) the occlusion effect.

Venting is done by creating a space between the CHA or ear mold and the ear canal. Kuk and Keenan[6] determined that widening the vent diameter by 1 mm decreases the objective occlusion effect by 4 dB. To fully avoid the occlusion effect, a vent diameter may have to be up to 5 mm. A large vent diameter required to eliminate the occlusion effect may not always be possible owing to space limitations (ie, a small ear canal). Open ear canal fittings, using a receiver-in-the-canal (RIC) CHA, which are extremely popular today are, in essence, a very well-vented or large vented CHA. This style is recommended to eliminate the occlusion effect for patients where the hearing loss at 500 Hz is 20 decibels hearing level or less.[6]

Although effective at decreasing, and even eliminating, the occlusion effect, venting, including through the use of open ear canal fittings, may not be appropriate for all patients. Venting size is often limited for patients with a significant high-frequency loss, because greater amplification is needed to maximize audibility, which often results in unwanted whistling, known as audible feedback. Therefore, venting may not be an option when there is a mild or moderate low-frequency hearing loss that slopes to a severe high-frequency hearing loss.[7] Another potential problem associated with venting is that it creates an open ear canal, allowing natural sound into the ear that is not affected by the CHA's signal processing. If natural sound dominates the amplified sound, the benefits of noise reduction and directional microphones are decreased.[5]

Another method to eliminate the occlusion effect is through deeper CHA canal fittings. Killion and associates[7] found that fitting the CHA or ear mold deep into the bony portion of the ear canal, close to the ear drum, decreases the occlusion effect by increasing impedance at the ear drum. Impedance at the ear drum increases the resonant frequency of the residual ear canal space and reduces the vibration of the ear canal.[7] Although they will relieve the occlusion effect, deep ear canal fittings have drawbacks in that they can be difficult for a clinician to fit and uncomfortable for a patient to wear. A deep ear canal fitting involves obtaining a deep ear mold impression. Some clinicians may be wary of obtaining a mold that must be close in proximity to the ear drum and the impression making process may cause patient discomfort. Deeply set CHA shells or ear molds are also often difficult to insert and remove. Finally, patients may find a deep fit uncomfortable, especially when worn for long periods of time.[5]

A way to lessen, but not eliminate, the undesirable consequences of the occlusion effect is to increase low-frequency gain. Although, as discussed elsewhere in this article, decreasing low-frequency gain is a method commonly touted for reducing the occlusion effect, increasing low-frequency gain is in fact the more effective approach. Added low-frequency gain allows the user to hear their own voice with amplified sound. This technique creates a better maintained consonant-to-vowel intensity ratio, which masks the annoyance of the occlusion effect and results in a more natural sound of one's own voice. Increasing low-frequency gain may have negative side effects, such as decreased sound quality and reduced ability to understand speech in situations where there is background noise.[6]

The skilled clinician must properly identify the occlusion effect and can then successfully decrease and even eliminate it. Through the use of venting, deeper canal fittings, or increasing low-frequency gain, clinicians can improve the quality of a patient's own voice to a satisfactory level, but should be wary that it may open up other problems such as feedback, discomfort, and CHA usage difficulty. Solving for the occlusion effect could also lead to decreased CHA functionality in the form of (1) less effective noise reduction, (2) reduced benefits of directional microphones, and (3) an overall decrease in sound quality.

Occlusion and Contralateral Routing of Signals

For traditional contralateral routing of signals (CROS) hearing aids, the user wears a microphone on the impaired ear, which is embedded into a behind-the-ear (BTE) or custom, in-the-ear (ITE), style CHA case. The microphone wirelessly transmits a signal to the hearing ear via a CHA. The CROS hearing aid is effective for providing 2-sided (but not true stereo) hearing, but the presence of a device in the better ear could lead to the occlusion effect. In those circumstances, an OI can be placed on the impaired side to pick up and then deliver sound directly to the hearing ear's cochlea via bone conduction, a process that avoids a device in the good ear and therefore presents no risk for occlusion.

Once they were introduced and approved, OIs were preferred over CROS hearing aids in the SSD population, in many cases owing to better performance and sound quality in noisy environments.[8–10] With improvement in CROS technology (eg, digital noise reduction and directional microphones), recent studies have shown that modern CROS hearing aids and OI users receive similar objective benefits from both devices.[11,12] Subjectively, Finbrow and colleagues[12] (2015) found that sound quality was superior in CROS hearing aids; 4 of their 8 participants preferred CROS hearing aids over OIs. Three preferred OIs based on nonsound quality factors, such as a preference for wearing one device instead of the 2 required in the CROS hearing aids and retention issues with the CROS domes. One participant did not have an overall preference because he found the sound quality of the CROS favorable, but preferred the OI for comfort.[13]

Although improvements in CROS devices might make CROS hearing aids preferable for many patients, allowing them to avoid the surgical procedure required for an OI, occlusion can be problematic for CROS users. To minimize the occlusion effect caused by the CHA worn on the hearing ear, the CHA can be well-vented (for an ITE-style CHA) or be an open ear piece (eg, dome) for RIC- or BTE-style CHAs. However, occlusion effect problems may persist for patients with narrow or curvy ear canals, where the vent size must be limited, or in instances where the CHA receiver itself may occupy a significant portion of the ear canal, as is sometimes the case for RIC-style CHAs. In addition, for SSD patients, if the CHA is too occluding, it can attenuate the natural sound entering the hearing ear. Should the occlusion effect be problematic for an SSD patient using, or trying, a CROS hearing aid, an OI may be an effective alternative.

FEEDBACK

Historically, feedback has been a major complaint associated with CHAs. In 2000, MarkeTrak VI found that only 44% of CHA users were satisfied with the whistling/feedback/buzzing of their CHAs.[13] This whistling, or high-frequency tonal sound emitted by CHAs, is known as acoustic feedback. Acoustic feedback occurs when the amplified sound of the CHA leaks out of the ear canal and is picked up by the microphone and then passed through the CHA again. Acoustic feedback is almost always present in CHAs, but is not always audible. Feedback will only be audible if the output of the receiver that reaches the microphone exceeds the original input level, which produces the whistling sound.[6]

Three Traditional Approaches to Reducing Feedback

To reduce or eliminate audible feedback, one approach is to simply reduce the gain at the problematic frequencies. Reducing the gain, however, will cause underamplification and decrease audibility.[6] A second approach to reduce feedback is decreasing the amount of sound leakage from the ear canal, which is accomplished by decreasing the vent size or creating a tighter fit of the CHA shell or ear mold. Decreasing the amount of sound leakage increases the attenuation of the feedback path and, accordingly, the amount of audible feedback. Decreasing sound leakage, however, also has its drawbacks. Decreasing the vent size, or eliminating the vent completely, may result in the occlusion effect, which, as discussed elsewhere in this article, is another problem for patients with a CHA. Decreasing sound leakage by creating a tighter fit of the CHA shell or ear mold and/or lengthening the canal can also lead to physical discomfort for patients.[14] A third approach to decreasing audible feedback is to pick a style of CHA that has a greater distance between the microphone and the receiver. For instance, completely-in-the-canal CHA have a short distance between the microphone and receiver, whereas RIC CHAs or larger ITE style CHAs (eg, half-shell or full-shell) have a greater distance. An individual with a significant hearing loss, needing high levels of gain, would require a greater distance between the microphone and receiver, such as provided by large ITE-style or RIC-style CHAs. However, if an individual is physically uncomfortable with such style and prefers a small ITE style (eg, a completely-in-the-canal CHA), it may result in reduced usage. Fortunately, RIC CHAs are extremely popular today, making up almost three-quarters of CHA sales, and also happen to be the preferred style when trying to minimize feedback.[15]

Modern Advances in Conventional Hearing Aids Have Reduced Feedback

Advanced digital signal processing in modern day CHAs has, on its own, reduced audible feedback, making the traditional techniques for reducing feedback not as crucial for many patients. Modern CHAs have digital feedback suppression (DFS) that, when used appropriately by a clinician, effectively reduces, and often eliminates, acoustic feedback. The clinician often has control over the activation and/or strength of the DFS approach in the computer software.

In modern high-end CHAs, DFS allows an addition of 9 to 16 dB of gain around the feedback critical area of 2 to 4 kHz before feedback is audible, with the effectiveness varying among manufacturers.[16] In lower end products, feedback management capabilities may be less effective. The additional gain allowed by DFS before feedback is audible allows individuals with more significant hearing loss to be fit with smaller custom CHAs (ie, completely-in-the-canal CHA) or less occluding CHAs using an open-fit style or a larger vent.

Combining Digital Feedback Suppression with Traditional Approaches

Although DFS provides effective feedback reduction, the traditional approaches for decreasing feedback may still be required. Properly fitting CHA shells and ear molds and appropriate vent size will still be needed when DFS does not provide enough protection against feedback, which is most likely to be the case for patients with significant high-frequency hearing losses.[15] As noted elsewhere in this article, the tradeoff of providing a patient with closer fitting CHA shells or ear molds and smaller vents is the possibility of creating the occlusion effect or physical discomfort.

Feedback Persists with User Error

A persistent problem with CHAs in general is user error, which plagues feedback, particularly in those with severe hearing losses (for whom DFS has not eliminated the problem). With DFS, feedback can, in theory, be eliminated or reduced significantly in the clinic for even those patients with severe hearing losses by ensuring a tight fit of the CHA shell or ear mold and proper insertion into the ear. However, user error, in the form of improperly inserting the CHA, results in audible feedback. Despite the clinician counseling the user on proper insertion, many patients, especially those with dexterity and/or cognitive declines, may not achieve optimal CHA placement. Even patients with good dexterity may struggle with proper placement should they have especially narrow or curvy ear canals. Noncustom ear pieces (eg, domes that are commonly used today with RIC CHAs to maximize comfort) can work their way out of the ear throughout the day even with precise insertion.

OTHER COMMON CONVENTIONAL HEARING AID COMPLAINTS AND ISSUES THAT MAY BE SOLVED BY IMPLANTABLE DEVICES
Comfort and Retention

Ear mold or CHA shell fit and retention (ie, CHAs falling out of the ear) may be problematic for CHA users. A poor CHA fit may result in itchiness and irritation and, in turn, decreased CHA use. Retention, and the resulting frequent reinsertion, can similarly lead to itchiness, irritation, and decreased CHA use, including as a result of lost or damaged CHAs. Although many CHA users will adapt, and the bothersome sensation will pass, for others, it will persist. There are many techniques a clinician can use to alleviate the irritation. For open-fit style CHAs, the clinician can change the dome style and/or tip. The tube or wire may be too short or too long and require a clinician testing different sizes to find a depth that is comfortable for the patient. Changing manufacturers can also be beneficial, because the shape and size of the domes, receivers, wires, and/or tubes are physically different across manufacturers.

Poor-fitting molds are one of the most frequent causes of irritation in CHA users, necessitating that clinicians solve for CHA fit to improve patient comfort. Custom molds with large vents may enhance comfort for open-fit style CHA users by providing a more stable fit in the ear canal. Custom molds can also be made for closed fitting CHAs. A clinician can often improve a poor-fitting mold by making modifications in the office (eg, buffing) or by taking a new ear mold impression using a different technique (eg, open jaw or closed jaw) or a different material (eg, acrylic) to be sent to the manufacturer. Even simply applying lubrication on the mold may improve the comfort of a custom or noncustom CHA.[17] With trial, error, and patience, most fit-related complaints can be ameliorated. However, for patients who remain dissatisfied and are unable to tolerate a CHA, an implantable device may become the appropriate choice.

Allergies

Allergic reactions to ear molds materials are uncommon, but possible. Switching the ear mold material from one type (eg, acrylic, vinyl) to silicone solves the problem for the majority of patients. However, silicone ear molds can also be problematic for some users by being difficult to insert, especially for those with very soft ears, or providing too tight a fit. Silicone molds typically provide a tight fit in the ear, which may pose a tolerance (ie, discomfort) problem for some patients.[18] Decreasing the size of the ear mold, a logical solution to a tight fit, can, in turn, lead to retention issues or make the CHA susceptible to feedback. Of course, some patients may also be allergic to silicone itself. For those patients who are also allergic to, or struggle using, silicone-based ear molds, an implantable device may be an appropriate solution to an acrylic or vinyl allergy.

Promoting Infections

Occluding the ear canal with an ear mold or CHA shell can induce or sustain external or middle ear infections by causing or exacerbating humidity in the ear canal. CHAs are simply not recommended for patients with chronic drainage. Venting the ear mold or CHA shell, or using an open-fit style CHA, can decrease or eliminate the moisture build up in the ear canal. Although venting will make the ear less prone to infection, allowing air into the ear canal can cause sound to leak out, making the CHA susceptible to acoustic feedback.

Infections, and the drainage caused by them, in addition to being uncomfortable for patients, may make the CHA prone to device failure for those patients with ITE and RIC CHAs, because the receiver and other electric components are in the ear and can malfunction when exposed to moisture. BTE CHAs may be appropriate for patients prone to infection, and the accompanying drainage, because all the components of the device are behind the ear and the ear mold can be cleaned and disinfected. For patients who prefer the RIC-style CHA for cosmetic reasons, modern BTE CHAs can use a thin tube for a more conspicuous appearance. A BTE CHA, coupled with a dome for an open fit, will minimize occlusion as well. Although no electronic components are in the ear canal in a BTE-style CHA, moisture can build up in the tube (even thin tubes) and cause damage to the CHA. Open-fit style CHAs, especially when used with a BTE, may lessen the threat of creating or exacerbating infections and device failure; however, they also may occlude the ear canal and, accordingly, not be appropriate for patients suffering from chronic infections. Chronic infection can often be managed by careful CHA selection, but severe cases may be a reason for a patient to switch to an implantable device.

Amplifying Conductive and Mixed Hearing Losses

Historically, studies showed that patients with 25 to 30 dB air–bone gaps performed better with an OI than a CHA, leading researchers to conclude that speech perception was better with OIs than with CHAs. At the time the studies were performed, amplification of CHAs was reduced to avoid feedback, a problem that is less common in modern CHAs.[19,20] Wolf and colleagues[20] (2010) fit patients with mixed hearing losses with modern CHAs, including feedback suppression technology, that were able to provide adequate amplification with no audible feedback. The study by Wolf and colleagues determined that patients with mixed hearing losses and a severe air–bone gap (30–35 dB or greater) still do better with OIs compared with BTE-style CHAs, having better speech recognition and preferring the sound quality with acoustic feedback no longer explaining the preference for OIs. Based on these results, OIs should be considered for patients with a severe air–bone gap.[21]

For patients with a CHA with significant air–bone gaps, the prescribed gain and maximum output requirements of a CHA is different than for patients with a CHA with sensorineural hearing loss. Hearing losses with air–bone gaps typically require less compression than sensorineural hearing loss. A substantial hearing loss with a significant air–bone gap, requiring a considerable amount of gain, can make the CHA particularly susceptible to feedback and more so than a similar hearing loss in a patient, whose loss is sensorineural in nature. Accordingly, for those air–bone gap patients, an OI can be an appropriate solution to decrease audible feedback.

Substantial gain requirements for patients with an air–bone gap can also pose a CHA style issue. Smaller CHA styles, such as ITEs or RICs, may not provide enough power even at the maximum output to support a patient's needs, necessitating the use of power BTEs. However, the size and visibility of a power BTE-style CHA may not be desirable to some patients. Clinicians should be cautious not to placate a patient by choosing a CHA style that, although less visible, offers inadequate maximum pressure output capabilities for the patient's needs. Setting a CHA to its maximum capabilities can degrade the sound quality owing to the saturation of high input level of both speech and nonspeech inputs.[21] In such circumstances, where a patient needs, but wants to avoid, a power BTE-style CHA, an OI may be offered as a solution.

WHEN CONVENTIONAL HEARING AIDS CAN STILL BE EFFECTIVE AND WHEN CONVENTIONAL HEARING AIDS REACH THEIR LIMIT

The inverse relationship of troubleshooting occlusion effect and audible feedback has historically plagued the use of CHAs. To reduce the occlusion effect a clinician will often open the ear canal by venting or by using an open-fit style CHA. By opening the ear canal, the CHA user is then subject to audible feedback, because the open canal allows significant sound to leak out of the ear. To decrease feedback, a clinician can then reduce the vent size or create a tighter fit, but that results in possible occlusion effect. When ensuring a comfortable physical fit or venting the ear canal for medical reasons, the risk of occlusion or feedback may be exacerbated.

As seen with the data obtained from MarkeTrak 9, CHA satisfaction has increased dramatically in recent years. The advent of DFS, and its significant improvement in modern CHAs, has allowed for audible feedback reduction while allowing the ear canal to remain open (ie, not creating the occlusion effect). DFS has undoubtedly contributed to patient's high CHA satisfaction rate. Many patients with mild to moderate hearing loss, and sometimes even more severe hearing loss, are now able to be successfully fit with their preferred CHA style and a comfortably fitting device.

Even if modern CHAs are used properly, audible feedback may still plague those with more significant hearing losses. Those with near-normal low-frequency hearing loss and severe-to-profound high-frequency hearing loss may not be able to achieve a satisfactory reduction of the occlusion effect without adding audible feedback. To eliminate the whistling, the clinician may have to make gain reductions to the high frequencies, compromising audibility. With increased satisfaction of CHAs, as seen in MarkeTrak 9, and evidence that implantable devices and optimally fitted CHAs have similar functional gain and speech recognition improvements,[15] the competitive advantage of MEI for many patients with moderate to severe sensorineural hearing losses may be reduced. For patients with significant hearing losses, however, it may not always be possible to (1) achieve an acceptable balance between occlusion effect and feedback, (2) ensure feedback does not occur without significantly reducing gain/audibility, and (3) guarantee a good comfortable physical fit. For these patients, MEIs and/or OIs may be an excellent alternative to CHAs.

REFERENCES

1. Haynes DS, Young JA, Wanna GB, et al. Middle ear implantable hearing devices: an overview. Trends Amplif 2009;13(3):206–14.
2. Ashburn-Reed S. The first FDA-approved middle ear implant. Hearing J 2001; 54(8):47–8.
3. Abrams HB, Kihm J. An introduction to MarkeTrak IX: a new baseline for the hearing aid market. Hearing Review 2015;22(6):16.
4. Dillon H. Hearing aids. Sydney (Australia): Boomerang Press; 2012.
5. Ricketts T, Bentler RA, Muller HG. Essentials of modern hearing aids: selection, fitting, and verification. Sand Diego (CA): Plural Publishing; 2019.
6. Kuk F, Keenan D. How do vents affect hearing aid performance? Hearing Review 2006;13(2):34–42.
7. Killion MC, Wilber LA, Gudmundsen G. Zwislocki was right… A potential solution to the "hollow voice" problem. Otology & Neurotology 1988;39(1):14–7.
8. Niparko JK, Cox KM, Lustig LR. Comparison of the bone anchored hearing aid implantable hearing device with contralateral routing of offside signal amplification in the rehabilitation of unilateral deafness. Otol Neurotol 2003;24:73–8.
9. Boseman AJ, Hol MK, Snik AF, et al. Bone-anchored hearing aids in unilateral inner ear deafness. Acta Otolaryngol 2003;123:258–60.
10. Lin LM, Bowditch S, Anderson MJ, et al. Amplification in the rehabilitation of unilateral deafness: speech in noise and directional hearing effects with bone-anchored hearing and contralateral routing of signal amplification. Otol Neurotol 2006;27:172–82.
11. Snapp HA, Hoffer ME, Liu Z, et al. Effectiveness in rehabilitation of current wireless CROS technology in experienced bone-anchored implant users. Otol Neurotol 2017;38:1397–404.
12. Finbow J, Bance M, Aiken S, et al. A comparison between wireless CROS and bone-anchored hearing devices for single-sided deafness: a pilot study. Otol Neurotol 2015;36:819–25.
13. Kochkin S. MarkeTrak VI: consumers rate improvements sought in hearing instruments. Otology & Neurotology 2002;9(11):18–22.
14. Chung K. Challenges and recent developments in hearing aids: part I. Speech understanding in noise, microphone technologies and noise reduction algorithms. Trends Amplif 2004;8(3):83–124.
15. US hearing aid sales Up 5.7% in first quarter 2018. Hearing Review 2018. Available at: http://www.hearingreview.com/2018/04/us-hearing-aid-sales-5-7-first-quarter-2018/. Accessed June 8, 2018.
16. Herbig R, Lueken C. A comparison of feedback cancellation systems in premier hearing aids. Hearing Review 2018;25(4):20–3.

17. Cui T. When hearing aids cause itchy ears, what can be done? Tao Cui. AudiologyOnline 2014. Available at: https://www.audiologyonline.com/ask-the-experts/when-hearing-aids-cause-itchy-12800. Accessed June 8, 2018.
18. West M. Earmolds and more: maximizing patient satisfaction Michael West. AudiologyOnline 2010. Available at: https://www.audiologyonline.com/articles/earmolds-and-more-maximizing-patient-850. Accessed June 8, 2018.
19. Mylanus EAM, van der Pouw CTM, Snik AFM, et al. Intraindividual comparison of the bone-anchored hearing aid and air-conduction hearing aids. Arch Otolaryngol Head Neck Surg 1998;124:271–6.
20. Wolf MJFD, Hendrix S, Cremers CWRJ, et al. Better performance with bone-anchored hearing aid than acoustic devices in patients with severe air-bone gap. Laryngoscope 2010;121(3):613–6.
21. Johnson EE. Prescriptive amplification recommendations for hearing losses with a conductive component and their impact on the required maximum power output: an update with accompanying clinical explanation. J Am Acad Audiol 2013;24(6):452–60.

Extended-Wear Hearing Technology
The Nonimplantables

Neil M. Sperling, MD[a,b,*], Scott E. Yerdon, AuD[c],
Marc D'Aprile, ScD, CCC-A[c]

KEYWORDS

- Lyric • Earlens • Extended-wear • Hearing aid • Nonimplantable

KEY POINTS

- A category of hearing technology has developed that consists of a deep ear canal device that remains in place for an extended period of time.
- These devices do not require a surgical event; they are inserted but not implanted.
- The ultimate goal of all hearing technologies is to improve auditory function with minimal discomfort, ease of application, and satisfactory cosmetics; a device that can meet these demands, while not requiring surgery for insertion, may be a preferred option.
- The extended-wear technologies offer distinct advantages to standard amplification.

 Video content accompanies this article at http://www.oto.theclinics.com.

INTRODUCTION

As the evolution of hearing technologies simultaneously pursues improvements in sound quality and delivery method, a category of hearing technology has developed that consists of a deep ear canal device that remains in place for an extended period of time. These devices do not require a surgical event; they are inserted but not implanted. In this sense, they represent an intermediate step in the continuum from hearing aid to implantable device. The ultimate goal of all hearing technologies is to improve auditory function with minimal discomfort, ease of application, and

Disclosure: All authors are providers of Earlens technology in a practice deemed a "Center of Excellence" by Earlens. They have not received compensation for this relationship.
[a] Department of Otolaryngology Head and Neck Surgery, New York Otolaryngology Group, Weill Cornell Medical College, 36A East 36th Street, New York, NY 10016, USA; [b] Departetnt of Otolaryngology, SUNY Downstate College of Medicine, 450 Clarkson Rd., Brooklyn, NY 11203, USA; [c] New York Otolaryngology Group, 36A East 36th Street, New York, NY 10016, USA
* Corresponding author. New York Otolaryngology Group, Weill Cornell Medical College, 36A East 36th Street, New York, NY 10016.
E-mail address: neil.sperling@nyogmd.com

Otolaryngol Clin N Am 52 (2019) 221–230
https://doi.org/10.1016/j.otc.2018.11.003
0030-6665/19/© 2018 Elsevier Inc. All rights reserved.

oto.theclinics.com

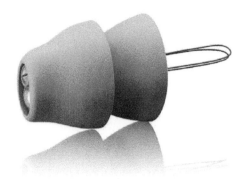

Fig. 1. Lyric device. (*Courtesy of* Sonova USA Inc, Warrenville, IL.)

satisfactory cosmetics. A device that can meet these demands, although not requiring surgery for insertion, may be a preferred option.

Over the past 2 decades, evolution in hearing aid systems sought to eliminate the recognized shortcomings of its technology. This included eliminating feedback and the occlusion effect, improving overall sound quality and hearing in noise, as well as addressing the lifestyle limitations of hearing aid use. Although many of these issues have improved with current hearing aid technology, some remain. The extended-wear technologies offer distinct advantages to standard amplification. Close proximity to the tympanic membrane (TM) and auditory anatomy appears to benefit patients using Lyric device. Earlens (Menlo Park CA, USA) has extended the audible bandwidth to 10 kHz, resulting in enhanced quality of sound significantly beyond that of standard amplification.

LYRIC

Lyric (Phonak AG, Stafa, Switzerland) was the first extended-wear hearing device, originally introduced in 2007. The device is inserted deeply into the ear canal by a hearing-instrument professional, a simple office-based nonsurgical procedure without

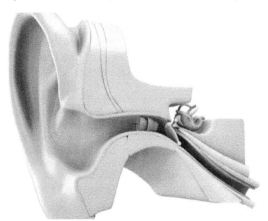

Fig. 2. Graphic of the Lyric device when deeply inserted into the ear canal. Note its proximity to the TM. Insertion and placement of Lyric should be 4 mm from the TM. (*Courtesy of* Sonova USA Inc, Warrenville, IL.)

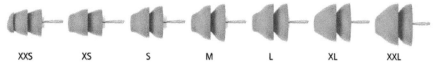

Fig. 3. Lyric devices and sizes. It is 12 mm in length. L, large; M, medium; S, small; XL, extra large; XS, extra small; XXL, extra extra large; XXS, extra extra small. (*Courtesy of* Sonova USA Inc, Warrenville, IL.)

anesthesia[1] (**Fig. 1**). The primary benefits of this device are related to its aesthetics and convenience. As such, this device appeals particularly to those concerned about wearing a visible device. In addition, it has advantages in disabled individuals or those unable to manipulate small devices.

By design, the device is placed into the bony portion of the ear canal 4 mm from the TM, minimizing the effect of cerumen and migrating exfoliated skin in the cartilaginous portion of the canal (**Fig. 2**). The device can be worn for up to 4 months, although replacement needs may vary by individual (eg, excessive cerumen production). Size is selected based on the ear canal dimensions (**Fig. 3**).

Lyric was first introduced by InSound Medical (Newark, CA, USA), which was later acquired by Sonova AG (Switzerland) in 2010. Lyric has gone through several iterations (Lyric, Lyric 2, and currently, Lyric 3), along with progressive change in its feature set. In May 2010, the Food and Drug Administration (FDA) recalled roughly 2000 Lyric 2 devices that were made in December 2009 due to a manufacturing error that could cause leakage from the battery.[2] This recall was terminated in August 2011.

Candidacy

Lyric is designed for mild to moderately severe hearing loss (**Fig. 4**). Candidacy for the Lyric device is dependent on good general health and absence of external ear disease or ongoing infectious middle ear disease. Other considerations include the size of the user's ear and the microbiology of the user's ear canal.[2] Individuals with uncontrolled diabetes, prior irradiation to the head and neck, immunodeficiency, age under 21 years, and/or those receiving anticoagulation therapy should be closely followed.[3] The Lyric is contraindicated in patients with TM perforations, chronic otorrhea, chronic ear infections, prominent osteoma or exostoses, pressure-equalizing tubes, or a history of cholesteatoma.

Design

There are 3 design aspects that enable the Lyric to be used for an extended time: (1) radial pressure on the skin of the canal, (2) breathability, and (3) placement. The device does not exceed the venous capillary pressure (20 mm Hg) by using a hydrophilic and flexible umbrella foam in order to allow for proper blood flow in the ear canal skin.[1] It uses open cell foam for moisture vapor transport as well as pressure equalization. Last, the device is ideally placed into the bony portion of the canal to prevent any effect on the sloughing of skin, to prevent irritation, and to reduce movement, all more likely in the cartilaginous portion of the canal. Of note, the device is water resistant but not waterproof, and therefore, the user is advised to avoid excessive water exposure, that is, swimming under water, but they may shower without ear protection.

Performance

Aesthetics and convenience are the prime motives for selecting a Lyric device. Lyric not only provides an individual the ability to "forget" about the repetitive insertion and removal of hearing devices but also eliminates the need to change batteries

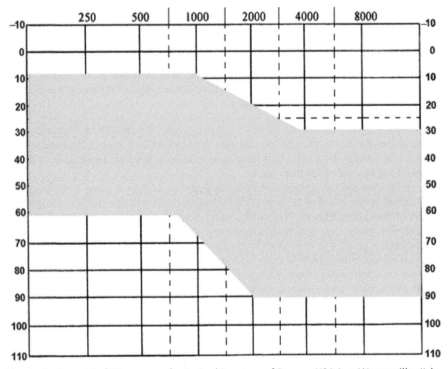

Fig. 4. Audiometric fitting range for Lyric. (*Courtesy of* Sonova USA Inc, Warrenville, IL.)

and provide wear and tear maintenance, including dehumidification, compared with conventional hearing instruments.

From an acoustical perspective, the amount of gain delivered by the Lyric device also differs from standard hearing aids. Typically, the further away from the TM the receiver is, the greater the amount of gain is required to correct an individual's hearing loss. Because the Lyric is closer to the TM, the gain required is not as great; this can reduce the risk of another common complaint of hearing aid wearers, feedback. In addition, the deep insertion of the Lyric device allows for the pinna to provide natural acoustic cues, such as aiding in localization.

Sound quality is an important aspect of all hearing devices. A field study sponsored by Phonak showed overall improvements in speech clarity, natural sound, and acceptance with Lyric 3 compared with Lyric 2.[4] These improvements in the Lyric 3 are related to the improved circuitry and phone use features.

The aesthetics of Lyric can have a positive psychosocial impact on the user. According to the manufacturer, compared with individuals who wear conventional air-conduction hearing aids, individuals wearing Lyric noted improvements in positive self-report.[5] Patient-reported improvements also included not having to worry about constant maintenance or tending to the device. In addition, the device sits securely in the ear, reducing the risk of losing the device, compared with traditional hearing aids.

Although Lyric is digitally programmable, it is an analog hearing aid. As such, there are limitations in terms of the digital signal processing that can be had. The analog components limit some of the desirable features found in other digital hearing aids, such as ear-to-ear communication, which enhances localization ability, along with more technologically savvy perks, such as Bluetooth and other connectivity capabilities.

Safety

A small percentage of Lyric users present with ear complications in which the device should be removed to allow for healing and on occasion referral for otolaryngology evaluation and treatment. Most commonly seen are abrasions, bleeding, ulcers, and otitis externa. The complications tend to occur in the first 2 weeks of placement and are a result of traumatic insertion, sizing error, poor placement, or patient manipulation of the device. In addition, the patient is counseled by the dispensing audiologist that if the device "dies" in their ear canal, they are to use the provided extraction tool and remove the device immediately. A retained Lyric in the ear canal for a prolonged time may lead to infection. An article published by Phonak indicated there have not been any incidents reported to the Lyric Quality Systems team of more serious complications, such as persistent TM perforation, osteomyelitis, or stenosis.[1] A publication by Thompson and colleagues[3] reports a rare case of benign necrotizing otitis externa/external ear canal cholesteatoma that was seen after Lyric placement.

Summary

Considering the aesthetic advantage and reduced care routine, Lyric devices may be advantageous for specific populations. Individuals with mild to moderately severe hearing loss who have normal ear anatomy and no ear/general health contraindications could be considered for this device. The proximity to the TM enhances reported sound quality, makes use of the external ear anatomy for localization, and reduces the likelihood of acoustic feedback.

Despite the ease of use of Lyric, this device has some detriments that the practitioner and user should take into consideration before proceeding. Some areas not widely discussed in the literature include limitations related to analog signal processing, restricting certain activities while wearing Lyric (eg, underwater swimming is not recommended), and lack of access to connectivity solutions. Last, because it is removed and replaced at 3- to 4-month intervals or sooner, the long-term cost of this device may be greater than most conventional air-conduction hearing aids.

EARLENS

In 1996, Dr Rodney Perkins[6] introduced the Earlens as a new method of transmitting sound to the human ear. This original report introduced several new concepts, including the feasibility of placing a transducer directly on the TM for an extended period of time. It also addressed several of the recognized shortcomings of standard amplification, including feedback, occlusion effect, and sound quality. The initial system involved an electromagnetic "collar" worn around the neck. A commercially available, solely ear-based, FDA-approved device was introduced in 2016.

The system uses a light-activated microactuator in contact with the umbo portion of the TM (**Fig. 5**). The microactuator is supported in place by a ring-shaped platform that includes a light detector and sits in the annular sulcus of the TM. An open-fit ear canal light tip is connected to a behind-the-ear (BTE) photon processor. Sound is processed and communicated to the light tip, which converts it to an invisible light emission. The emitted light is detected by the photo detector on the TM lens, which converts it to mechanical movement of the actuator on the umbo, augmenting the natural auditory physiology. Direct umbo stimulation produces less acoustic feedback than traditional

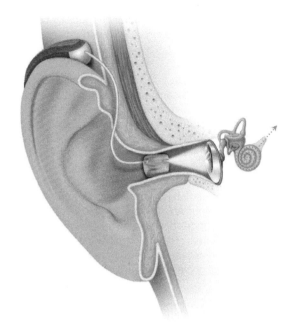

Fig. 5. Graphic of Earlens system in place. (*Courtesy of* Earlens Co, Menlo Park, CA.)

acoustic amplification at equivalent frequency amplitudes and leads to enhanced high-frequency gains (125–10,000 Hz) without feedback.[7]

Candidacy

Individuals with mild to severe hearing loss can be considered for Earlens fitting (**Fig. 6**). The ear canal must accommodate lens insertion, eliminating individuals with narrow canals or exostoses. An intact TM is required. This device has not been used in individuals who have a history of middle ear disease or prior ear surgery.

Design

Earlens consists of 3 main components: the *BTE Photon Processor*, which is connected to the ear canal; the *Light Tip*, which communicates wirelessly with the *Tympanic Lens* (**Fig. 7**). The lens is custom made according to the patient's anatomy, based on deep ear canal impressions. The lens consists of a platform that conforms to the patient's tympanic sulcus. A coating of mineral oil and the lens' customized shape keep it in position. Its open design and layer of oil allow for natural egress of epithelium and keratin.

The lens is constructed of a form-fitting perimeter platform that conforms to the annular sulcus. It also supports the moving parts that transmit the signal at the umbo platform.

Impressions

Deep ear canal impressions required for Earlens fitting may be new to the dispensing audiologist or hearing instrument specialist, because there is no foam otoblock between the impression mold and the TM. Given that the impression includes the TM surface, it is the otolaryngologist who is appropriately equipped for this procedure. Microscopic and endoscopic views of the medial ear canal and annular sulcus are

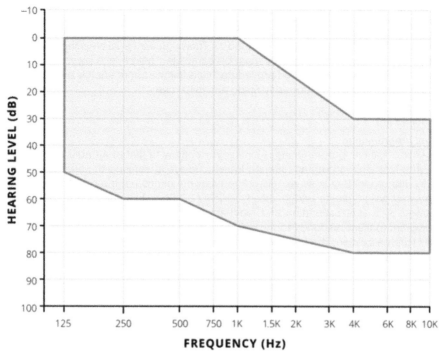

Fig. 6. Audiometric fitting range for Earlens. (*Courtesy of* Earlens Co, Menlo Park, CA.)

important to obtaining the optimal fit. Under microscopic guidance, and with familiar instrumentation, the otolaryngologist can comfortably work at the TM surface without adverse event.

The impression procedure uses 2 impression materials separated in time and patient position. A low-viscosity deep impression of the TM and bony ear canal is completed as the patient is in the supine position. A successive higher-viscosity impression of the lateral ear canal and conchal area is done in the sitting position. After the cure time is completed, the composite impression is mobilized and removed by hand. No anesthesia is required. At the moment that the impression breaks its seal with the TM/ear canal, there may be brief discomfort. This procedure takes approximately 15 minutes for each ear and generally is tolerated well.

Impressions are used to build a custom-fit lens and light tip and to assure proper alignment of the 2.

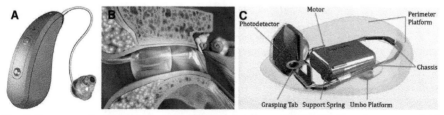

Fig. 7. Components of Earlens system: (*A*) photon processor, (*B*) light tip in the ear canal, (*C*) lens. (*Courtesy of* EarLens Corporation, Menlo Park, CA.)

Insertion

Once the customized lens and light tip/processor are available, the otolaryngologist places the lens onto the TM (**Fig. 8**, Video 1). Thorough ear canal cleaning and application of a thin layer of mineral oil must be completed before lens placement. Lens placement is a brief office-based procedure that is followed immediately by audiologic programming to provide same-day fitting and initial use.

Programming

Initial programming

In general, Earlens programming is similar in workflow to that of a traditional hearing aid. The first step in programming an Earlens device is entering the audiogram into "ELF," the proprietary software. Step 2 requires connection of the photon processor to a wired programming bridge called "HI-PRO 2." Step 3 is detection of the device followed by a light calibration and feedback test. Light calibration is similar to an audiogram (patient responds to the softest audible pure tone) from 0.125 to 10 kHz. After light calibration, the feedback test eliminates any possibility of acoustic feedback. In the final step, step 4, the data are saved to the photon processor and the aids are disconnected from the HI-PRO 2 cables.

There are exceptions to the rules above. After step 3, if a patient is uncomfortable with the sound quality, the audiologist may adjust multiple parameters (including but not limited to pitch, maximum equivalent pressure output [MEPO], expansion, manual volume control, and listening algorithms). After all sound quality–related concerns are addressed, the devices are paired via low-energy Bluetooth with the patient's cell phone (currently only available on Apple products). This pairing allows for the patient to customize their listening experience while seamlessly streaming phone calls, music, and other audio.

First follow-up

The patient returns 1 week after their initial fitting. During this appointment, the audiologist addresses any patient questions or concerns. Otoscopy is completed to verify proper lens position. Last, the patient is tested functionally in a sound-treated booth with narrowband noise from 125 Hz to 10 kHz in the sound field. If any frequency response is more than 25 dB HL (hearing level), the devices are reprogrammed to be slightly louder at those specific frequencies.

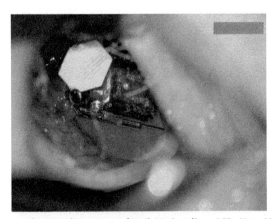

Fig. 8. Lens in situ on the TM. (*Courtesy of* Neil M. Sperling, MD, New York, NY.)

Subsequent follow-up

When all patient concerns have been addressed and hearing thresholds have been verified to be 25 dB or better from 0.125 to 10 kHz, the patient returns to clinic every 3 months (4 times per year) for verification of lens placement and professional cleaning of the light tip. The visit generally includes evaluation by the audiologist and otolaryngologist. The patient is encouraged to return if there are any issues between this time interval.

Performance

Data from the preliminary studies of Earlens revealed favorable safety measures and outcomes. Outcome measures included maximum outputs of 90 to 110 dB for frequencies up to 10 kHz, and maximal stable gain before feedback of more than 40 dB even at higher frequencies with a widely vented ear canal.[8,9] In general, studies on feedback of traditional amplification indicate the presence of feedback at far lower inputs.

Earlens delivers output to much higher frequencies than current hearing aids. At lower frequencies, Earlens MEPO would be comparable to traditional amplification less than 5500 Hz except that Earlens also adds an extension of low-frequency amplification to 125 Hz, whereas traditional amplification does not typically go below 500 Hz.

TM damping was the measured effect of the lens on hearing without amplification. The mean overall TM damping across all frequencies was 4.1 dB. A slight fullness in the ear is commonly reported with the lens in place but is not noticed when the device is active.

MEPO is a measure of output at the point of contact with the TM that corresponds to the maximum pressure outputs of an acoustic hearing aid. MEPO is used as a measure of maximal output of an Earlens device. Maximum outputs for Earlens, as measured in a 2016 temporal bone study, were 120 to 136 dB sound pressure level.[9]

From the clinical study published in 2017, impressive outcome measures include average word recognition improvement of 33% compared with unaided condition, an average functional gain of 30 dB from 2 to 10 Hz, and maximal functional gain of 68 dB at 9 and 10 kHz.[7]

These findings imply significant benefit to patients with hearing loss, including those who would otherwise be considered poor traditional hearing aid candidates.

As noted in Gantz and colleagues,[7] the functional gains achieved with Earlens compares favorably with some implanted devices and exceeds them at high frequencies.

Maintenance

The Earlens system requires patient maintenance, including instillation of oil in the ear several times per week. The oil maintains a layer between the lens and TM, allowing epithelial migration to continue uninterrupted. The lens is designed to remain in place for months to years.

Safety

Only mild temporary adverse effects from this system have been reported and included ear canal discomfort, abrasion, or swelling. In the safety study published in 2017, all such effects resolved except for ear fullness that was reported in 1 of 41 patients.[7] TM injury has not been reported. None of the reported adverse events were considered serious.

Summary

Earlens appears to be a significant advance in hearing technology. The physics of light energy in the ear canal avoids some of the limitations of acoustically based amplification. The extension of functional gain to low and high frequencies enhances subjective sound quality. This extension of audible frequencies is likely to add clarity and enhance hearing in noise. The available data are promising. Long-term data are not yet available.

SUPPLEMENTARY DATA

Supplementary data related to this article can be found online at https://doi.org/10.1016/j.otc.2018.11.003.

REFERENCES

1. Johnson J. Clinical and medical review. Phonak Field Study News 2015;1–6. Available at: https://www.accessdata.fda.gov/scripts/cdrh/cfdocs/cfRes/res.cfm?ID=88543.
2. Biggins A, Solodar H. Healthy ears for Lyric wearers – the contributing key factors. Phonak Field Study News 2017;1–4.
3. Thompson C, Gohil R, Bennett A, et al. Lyric hearing aid: a rare cause of benign necrotizing otitis externa/external ear canal cholesteatoma. BMJ Case Rep 2017. https://doi.org/10.1136/bcr-2017-222719.
4. Banerjee S. In support of Lyric3. Phonak Field Study News 2016;1–4.
5. Biggins A, Singh G, Solodar H. Lyric shows significant psychosocial benefits. Phonak Field Study News 2017;1–6.
6. Perkins R. Earlens tympanic contact transducer: a new method of sound transduction to the human ear. Otolaryngol Head Neck Surg 1996;114:720–8.
7. Gantz BJ, Perkins R, Murray M, et al. Light-driven contact hearing aid for broad-spectrum amplification: safety and effectiveness pivotal study. Otol Neurotol 2017;38:352–9.
8. Fay JP, Perkins R, Levy SC, et al. Preliminary evaluation of a light-based contact hearing device for the hearing impaired. Otol Neurotol 2013;34:912–21.
9. Puria S, Santa Maria PL, Perkins R. Temporal-bone measurements of the maximum equivalent pressure output and maximum stable gain of a light-driven hearing system that mechanically stimulates the Umbo. Otol Neurotol 2016;37:160–6.

Physiology of Osseointegration

Jennifer Wing Yee Lee, BSc(Med), MBBS, MS, FRACS*,
Manohar Lal Bance, MB ChB, MSc, FRCSC, FRCS

KEYWORDS

- Bone conduction implant • Conductive hearing loss • Single-sided deafness
- Osseointegration • Titanium • Osseoimmunology

KEY POINTS

- Bone conduction implant devices rely on osseointegration, which create a structural interface between titanium implant surface and bone of the underlying skull.
- Osseointegration incorporates processes in the initial tissue response to implantation: peri-implant osteogenesis and peri-implant bone remodeling, which ultimately lead to de-novo bone formation on the implant surface.
- Osseointegration is immune-mediated, driven by the complement system and macrophages and characterized by tissue reparative features.
- Implant design, composition, and surface topography modifications can enhance osseointegration.
- Other factors that affect osseointegration include patient local and systemic factors, surgical technique, adequate healing time, and loading characteristics.

INTRODUCTION

Bone conduction implant devices (BCIDs) are indicated in the auditory rehabilitation of patients with conductive or mixed hearing loss who are unable to wear traditional hearing aids or for patients with single-sided deafness. The first implantation of BCIDs was in 1977 by Anders Tjellstrom[1] and since then, there have been more than 200,000 recipients of BCIDs worldwide.

BCIDs rely on osseointegration with the skull, the process of creating a structural and functional interface between the surface of a load-bearing bioactive implant and living bone, without intervening soft tissue.[1,2] The aim is to achieve endosseous healing and to induce de-novo bone formation surrounding and directly onto the implant surface, which prevents any further relative movement between implant and

Disclosure: The authors have no disclosures or commercial or financial conflicts of interest.
Otology and Skull Base Unit, Cambridge University Hospitals NHS Foundation Trust, Hills Road, Cambridge CB20QQ, UK
* Corresponding author.
E-mail address: jennifer.w.lee@hotmail.com

bone under normal conditions of loading. Intimate bone apposition to the implant material generates improved stability, decreased risk of failure, and creates implant longevity. Ideally, vibrations generated by the device are transmitted efficiently to the bone without loss.

The term "osseointegration" was coined by Per-Ingvar Brånemark of Sweden, after he observed this process occurring with titanium implants in rabbit bones.[3] The implant titanium oxide layer became permanently incorporated within the bone, such that the 2 could not be separated without fracture. The concept of osseointegration today can be studied clinically, anatomically, histologically, and ultrastructurally.[4]

Most of our understanding about osseointegration in-vivo comes from experience with dental implants and limb prostheses but while these are often made of alloys, manufacturers of BCIDs have favored pure titanium compositions. Apart from high tensile strength, the titanium oxide layer provides corrosion resistance and has excellent biocompatibility, being nontoxic to macrophages and fibroblasts.[5] In addition, the oxide layer has the ability to repair itself by reoxidation when damaged. The surface characteristics of implants may also be altered to enhance osseointegration or shorten the time taken for bone fixation.

STAGES OF OSSEOINTEGRATION

The stages of osseointegration[4] are as follows:

- Initial tissue response to implantation
- Peri-implant osteogenesis
- Peri-implant bone remodeling

Initial Tissue Response to Implantation

The initial stage of osseointegration commences with drilling the implant socket within the bone followed by inserting the titanium implant into the bed. Immediately after surgical insertion, primary implant stability is from passive mechanical apposition and engagement between implant and bone. Cortical bone is preferable to cancellous bone for primary stability. Meticulous surgical technique is important, including the use of copious cooling irrigation solution and low speed drilling. Subjecting titanium implants to a temperature elevation of 47°C for 1 minute can cause bone necrosis.[6]

The trauma of implant placement and injury to the underlying bone generate an inflammatory response characterized by release of growth factors and cytokines that form an extracellular matrix and hematoma for bone repair.[2,7] Within the clot, platelets undergo a cascade of adhesion and aggregation and the resultant fibrin matrix serves as a scaffold for migration (osteoconduction), proliferation, and differentiation (osteoinduction) of leukocytes and mesenchymal cells from post-capillary venules to the peri-implant site.[4,8,9] This process occurs within 1 to 3 days after surgical implantation.

Peri-Implant Osteogenesis

During the first 7 days, angiogenesis takes place within the peri-implant gap,[10] and from day 1 to around 2 weeks, the mesenchymal cells differentiate into osteoblasts, which form a cell-rich, immature, woven bone through intramembranous ossification.[10] The mesenchymal cells produce a 0.5-mm thick afibrillar, noncollagenous extracellular matrix layer, rich in calcium, phosphorus, osteopontin, and bone sialoprotein,[11] on the implant surface. There is a separate 20 to 50 mm layer of osteoblast-like cells, calcified collagen fibrils, and early mineralization at the implant-bone interface.[12] Woven bone continues to form over 2 weeks after implantation, with the implant surface acting as a biomimetic scaffold.[13]

Marrow tissue with its rich vasculature supports the mesenchymal cells and provides precursors of osteoclasts. Woven bone has low mechanical competence due to random orientation of collagen fibers but from about day 10, the rapidly formed trabecular bone with its bridgelike architecture provides early active biological fixation of the implant. This optimally occurs when the gap between implant and bone does not exceed 500 μm. The valley regions of threaded implants are believed to be associated with increased bone formation kinetics.

Peri-Implant Bone Remodeling

Osteoclasts drive the process of bone resorption and remodeling of the woven bone and replacement by lamellar bone with a higher degree of mineralization. Titanium induces the host to favor bony remodeling over resorption. The osteoclasts attach to the mineralized collagen matrix, forming a sealing zone, depositing bone directly onto the implant surface. Lamellar bone allows adaptation to a greater load, with bone fibers deposited in parallel formation and new osteons circling around the implant with their long axes perpendicular to the long axis of the implants. This provides active secondary fixation of the implant through biological bonding.[14] At 3 months post-implantation, a mixed texture of woven and lamellar bone can be found around titanium implants, whereas the late stage of osseointegration can take a year or longer to complete. During this time, on the implant side, oxidation of the titanium is observed.

In the area up to 1 mm of bone from the implant surface, there is a continual dynamic process of remodeling in response to stress and mechanical loading months to years following implantation. This is confirmed by the long-term presence of marrow spaces containing osteoclasts, osteoblasts, mesenchymal cells, and vascular tissue next to the implant surface.

The degree of stability achieved by osseointegration is more important than the actual degree of contact between the surfaces, measured by bone-implant contact (BIC) percentage. Failure of osteogenesis can occur due to[4] the following:

- Decreased number and/or activity of osteogenic cells
- Increased osteoclastic activity
- Imbalance between anabolic and catabolic factors on bone formation
- Micromotion of the implant or mechanical stress leading to osteolysis
- Impaired vascularization of peri-implant tissue

Excessive implant micromotion during healing results in tensile and shear motions, stimulating a fibrous membrane formation around the implant and causing displacement at the bone-implant interface. This can cause aseptic loosening, inhibition of osseointegration, and implant loss. In a canine study, 20 μm of oscillating displacement was compatible with stable bone ingrowth, whereas 40 and 150 μm of motion were not tolerated and led to exuberant bone formation in the bone-implant gap.[15]

OSTEOIMMUNOLOGY

Early research focused on the role of osteoblasts and osteoclasts in osseointegration. More recently, there is increasing evidence that osseointegration is in fact an immunologically driven process, relying on advantageous inflammatory pathways that promote de-novo bone formation as part of the host response to bioactive implants, and reducing the negative tissue responses that could lead to rejection.[16,17] Titanium implants are classified as bioactive implants, which have the ability to drive inflammation and differ to chemically inert implants that merely elicit a short-lived foreign body response that results in fibrous encapsulation. Studies have shown that application of nonsteroidal antiinflammatory drugs in animal models, which inhibit prostaglandins such as PGE2, led to inhibition of angiogenesis and osseointegration.[18,19] The main driving force for osteoimmunology is the host innate immunity, particularly the complement cascade and macrophage activation.

Macrophages are the major effector cell in immune reactions to biomaterials, controlling inflammation, healing, and even long-term response to different stimuli. Monocytes and macrophages are abundant in bone marrow and periosteal and endosteal tissues, where they are known as OsteoMacs,[16,20] and they regulate tissue homeostasis and provide immune surveillance. OsteoMacs constitute approximately one-sixth of all cells residing in bone marrow. OsteoMacs release bioactive growth factors such as tumor necrosis factor α,[21] transforming growth factor β,[22] interleukins 6 and 1,[23,24] osteopontin,[25] 1,25-dihydroxy-vitamin D3,[26] and BMP-2,[27] which induce extracellular matrix deposition and facilitate neoosteogenesis. Macrophages can be classified into 2 specific cell types: classic M1 proinflammatory macrophages that facilitate osteoclastogenesis and M2 tissue reparative macrophages.[17,28] The M2 phenotype is thought to be dominant in osseointegration.

Knockout models have demonstrated that removal of OsteoMacs from in vitro cultures leads to a 23-fold decrease in osteogenic differentiation and mineralization.[20] In areas of bone modeling, OsteoMacs have been observed to encapsulate functionally mature osteoblasts and provide signals that dictate osteoblastic function. In knockout mice models, depletion of OsteoMacs can cause loss of endosteal osteoblasts, reduction of trophic cytokines at the endosteum, and a complete loss of bone modeling.[29]

Osteoclasts and osteoblasts maintain a steady state of bone formation and resorption. Bone remodeling provides the mechanism for adaptation to mechanical stress, repair of microdamage, and replacement of primary bone during osseointegration of implants. Macrophage precursors differentiate into osteoclasts under the influence of cytokines CSF1 and RANKL,[30,31] and their attachment and activation are mediated by integrins, particularly vitronectin receptor $\alpha V\beta 3$.[32] Attachment of $\alpha V\beta 3$ induces signaling mechanisms that control cytoskeletal reorganization.

Following implantation of biomaterial where the foreign particle is too large for macrophage phagocytosis, several macrophages under the influence of many different cytokines, including interleukin 4 and 13, fuse together to form multinucleated giant cells.[33] Research suggests giant cells around bony implants contribute more to tissue integration and wound healing than biomaterial rejection.[20,28,34] They can be identified at the surface of osseointegrated implants after many years, and it is postulated that chronic immune-mediated inflammation is present for the lifetime of the implant in the bone.

Implant failure due to bone loss is thought to be due to excessive bone resorption by osteoclasts. Furthermore, studies have shown that hydrophilic and anionic substrate surfaces cause less macrophage adherence, increased apoptosis, and decreased giant cell formation.

IMPLANT SURFACE CHARACTERISTICS

The literature reports that modification of the implant surface to increase roughness has a significant effect on favoring osseointegration.[35,36] Rough surfaces allow platelet and monocyte adhesion, enhancement of osteoblast attachment and subsequent proliferation and differentiation, and increase in surface area of implant in contact with the host bone. In addition, macrophage cell proliferation and adhesion, release of proinflammatory markers, and TGF-β and BMP-2 gene expression[37] are increased in implants with greater surface roughness. Lastly, surface roughness promotes M2 macrophage phenotype[38] and accelerates differentiation of macrophages into osteoclasts.[39]

Surface topography can be modified on multiple levels from macroscopic design or shape of implant, to introduction of microscopic, submicron, or nano-textures superimposed on one another. Surface roughness can be increased by machining, plasma spray coating (spraying titanium dissolved in heat onto the implant surface), grit blasting (spraying particles with ceramic or silica), acid etching (applying hydrofluoric, sulfuric, or nitric acid), sandblasting and acid etching, anodizing (applying voltage to breakdown the titanium oxide layer), or biomimetic coating.[40]

These modifications can create nanostructures of varying shapes on biomaterial surfaces, including porous, tubular, or pitlike shapes. The ideal dimension, aspect ratio, or distribution of nanostructures on implant surfaces to provide optimal functionality remains under intense research. Matching the implant surface characteristics to the hierarchical architecture of actual bone seems to provide ideal bioactive potential.[41]

Wennerberg and Albrektsson propose the following categories for surface roughness based on the surface area (Sa) value[41]:

- Smooth surfaces: Sa value less than 0.5 μm
- Minimally rough surfaces: Sa value 0.5 to less than 1.0 μm, include the Brånemark turned fixture
- Moderately rough surfaces: Sa value 1 to less than 2.0 μm, include the Astra Tech TiOblast and Osseospeed implants
- Rough surfaces: Sa value greater than or equal to 2 μm, include implant surfaces treated with plasma spray

In 2012, Cochlear introduced the Baha DermaLock (BA400) abutment on its percutaneous Baha Connect implants into clinical practice (Cochlear BAS, Mölnlycke, Sweden). This technology applies a hydroxyapatite coating on the concave-designed abutment surface, providing greater bioactivity and larger surface area than conventional titanium. The ceramic surface is purported to create better dermal adherence to the implant, thereby preventing downgrowth and migration of the overlying epidermis and allowing soft tissue preservation surgery.[42] This has been part of an evolution in surgical strategy world-wide in which there is less subdermal tissue reduction, and more preservation of full thickness tissues, which seem to decrease postoperative soft-tissue complications, decreased pain, less paraesthesia, shorter operative times, and better cosmesis.[43–45] Other possible advantages of hydroxyapatite coatings are faster osteoblast differentiation, enhanced biomechanics resulting in higher carrying loads, and increased bone penetration.

In a clinical review of 30 consecutive patients undergoing implant surgery using the Cochlear DermaLock (BA400) abutment, 86.7% of patients had no soft-tissue reactions, and mean time from implantation to processor loading was 4.5 weeks.[46]

The use of DermaLock is in addition to Cochlear's use of TiOblast titanium, with increased roughness at the actual bone interface. The TiOblast surface is manufactured with a physical subtractive procedure, by sandblasting the surface with spherical particles of titanium dioxide, and gives an Sa value of 1.1 μm.[47] In vivo tests demonstrate that the titanium dioxide particles, which carry negative charge, facilitate the deposition of calcium ions onto the implant, and stimulate the activity of osteoprogenitor cells to create more dense bony trabeculae (**Fig. 1**).

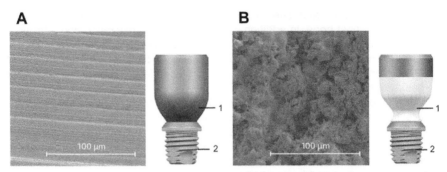

Fig. 1. Comparison between the Cochlear BA300 and Cochlear DermaLock BA400 abutments. The scanning electron microscopy images of their respective surfaces compare the surface topography of (*A*) a machined surface finish (BA300) and (*B*) a sandblasted finish with hydroxyapatite coating (BA400). (Image courtesy of Cochlear Bone Anchored Solutions AB, 2018.)

In 2015, Oticon Medical released their Ponto BHX implant, which combines Opti-Grip geometry and the Brånemark Biohelix surface modification (Oticon Medical AB, Askim, Sweden). The OptiGrip geometry refers to the gradual relieving behind the cutting edge of the implant, which means less tissue pressure and friction at time of implantation.[48] There is still a high bone-implant contact surface afforded by an increase in the threaded area along the length of the implant, which allows a smaller drill diameter at surgery while maintaining higher primary stability of the implant shortly following surgery.

The Biohelix surface is created by a micromachining process, where an oscillating laser beam is used to heat and ablate the titanium at the root or inner part of the thread of the abutment. This induces a nanoporous structure and roughness to the implant surface in a process that does not require addition of any chemicals.

In an animal model, laser-modified titanium screws had significantly higher biomechanical anchorage, as determined by removal torque measurements, compared with machined titanium screws.[49] The laser-modified screws had higher microroughness and increased surface titanium dioxide layer thickness. Histologic and electron microscopy analysis of the bone and extracellular matrix composition involved in the osseointegration process was similar between the 2 types of implants (**Fig. 2**).

Another BCID that relies on osseointegration is the BCI developed from collaboration between Chalmers University of Technology and Sahlgrenska University Hospital in Sweden. The device uses transcutaneous electromagnetic transduction of sound but the implanted component consists of a flat surface in contact with bone, rather than a screw-design implant. Despite the flat surface, preclinical and animal studies on sheep have demonstrated successful osseointegration of the implant, allowing comparable sound transmission to that achieved in percutaneous implants.[50] Further experimental implants have been described that may also exhibit osseointegration.

Currently studies are underway to evaluate the effects of many bioactive surface modifications, such as the addition of growth factors (bone morphogenetic proteins, osteogenic protein-1, insulinlike growth factor, transforming growth factor β, and fibroblast growth factor) and extracellular matrix components (collagen, chondroitin sulfate, fibronectin, and hyaluronic acid). The hypothesis is that these biocoatings may accelerate or enhance the quality of osseointegration, but so far early animal studies for dental implants with biological coatings have not shown any benefit.[51]

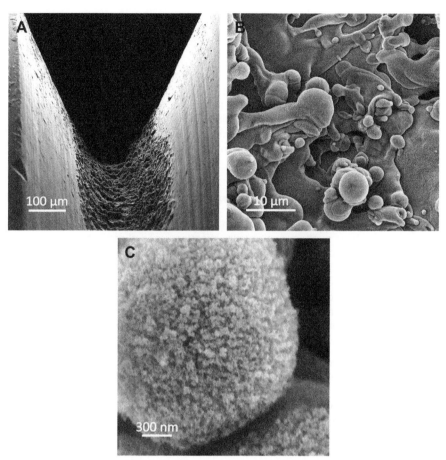

Fig. 2. The surface modifications on the Oticon Biohelix abutment surface at a (*A*) macroscopic, (*B*) microscopic, and (*C*) nanoscopic level. (With permission from Oticon Medical, 2017.)

LOADING AND CLINICAL ASSESSMENTS FOR OSSEOINTEGRATION

Conventional or delayed functional loading after implantation is designed to allow the titanium implant to complete healing and establish secondary stability in order to avoid micromotion of the implant. As outlined previously, early integration occurs within a few weeks after implantation, but the full process of osseointegration can take months. Early in the development of BCIDs, loading of an implant would only occur after at least 3 months of undisturbed healing time. However, much shorter delays in loading are now implemented in most centers, on the order of 2 to 4 weeks, without significant impact on implant failure rate.

Implant stability is an indirect indication of osseointegration and can be clinically assessed by various methods:

- Clinical mobility test
- Radiological imaging
- Resonance frequency analysis (RFA)

Radiological imaging is aimed at demonstrating direct contact between bone and implant, whereas radiolucency may indicate the presence of fibrous tissue at the bone-implant interface. Imaging resolution and lack of standardized radiographic reporting are limiting factors to its use.

An RFA device contains a piezoelectric element that induces oscillations and attaches to the implant and a probe that reads its corresponding resonance frequency. This frequency is translated into an implant stability quotient (ISQ), which ranges from 1 to 100, with 100 being the highest stability state. Exposed implant length, healing time, stiffness of the surrounding bone, implant geometry, and location of implant can affect the ISQ value. In addition, there are no established diagnostic threshold criteria available to guide clinical use.

FACTORS THAT AFFECT OSSEOINTEGRATION

Failure of osseointegration remains one of the main complications of BCIDs, in addition to skin problems such as overgrowth, infections, and allergy. Implant loss was recorded in 8.3% of patients in a study of more than 1000 percutaneous BCIDs,[52] with a meta-analysis reporting variable rates from 2% to 17%.[53] Higher rates are seen in the pediatric population and patients aged older than 60 years, thought to be due to less bone stock, reduced bone vascularity, and higher possibility of postoperative trauma to the abutment. Factors that may affect osseointegration both positively and negatively include the following:

- Implant factors: design, shape, length, diameter, composition and its biocompatability, surface macroscopic and microscopic topography and treatment, osteogenic biological coatings, surface energy and wettability, and implant micromotion;
- Host factors: implant bed site, bone cellularity and density (osteoporosis), intrinsic osteogenic potential, systemic illness (rheumatoid arthritis, smoking status, renal insufficiency, nutritional deficiency), medications (bisphosphonates, statins, immunosuppressants and steroids, cisplatinum, warfarin, heparins, nonsteroidal antiinflammatory drugs), and previous local radiotherapy;
- Surgical technique: minimal tissue injury, adequate clearance of soft tissue, continuous cooling, and low speed drilling may all enhance osseointegration;
- Undisturbed healing time and 2-stage surgical procedure (implant loading delayed until after submerged healing period) may be indicated in patients prone to poor osseointegration;
- Loading conditions: overloading may interfere with osseointegration.

From in vitro and animal studies, osteoporosis is associated with slower osseointegration and higher rate of implant failures.[54,55] Osteoporosis affects proliferation of mesenchymal cells, protein synthesis, and cell reactivity to local factors. Osteoblast numbers and activity are decreased, vascularity is impaired, and osteoclast numbers and activity are increased. Bisphosphonates that inhibit osteoclast-mediated bone resorption seem to enhance implant stability in patients with low bone density or metabolic bone diseases.[56,57]

The lipid-lowering statins are also believed to have an osteoanabolic effect. Histomorphometric studies have shown increased bone ingrowth, interface strength, implant stability, and osseous adaptation[58] in patients on these medications.

The effect of external beam radiation therapy on osseointegration remains unknown. Evidence suggests that it leads to delay in bone remodeling.[59] A study examined oral Brånemark implants retrieved from pre- or post-operatively irradiated sites[60] and reported that implants with shorter duration in situ had sparse osseointegration but implants with longer time in situ had high BIC up to 70%. It is thought that osseointegration can still be successful in areas receiving full doses of irradiation but there are overall higher rates of implant failure.

SUMMARY

BCIDs rely on osseointegration and immune-driven process that creates a structural interface between titanium implant surface and bone of the underlying skull. This phenomenon is characterized by de-novo peri-implant osteogenesis and bone remodeling and when complete, prevents further movement of the implant in relation to the underlying bone. Implant design and modification, host systemic and local factors, surgical technique, and loading conditions contribute to the success or failure of osseointegration.

REFERENCES

1. Tjellstrom A, Lindstrom J, Hallen O, et al. Osseointegrated titanium implant in the temporal bone: a clinical study on bone-anchored hearing aids. Am J Otol 1981; 2:304–10.
2. Lotz EM, Berger MB, Schwartx Z, et al. Regulation of osteoclasts by osteoblast lineage cells depends on titanium implant surface properties. Acta Biomater 2018;68:296–307.
3. Branemark PI. Vital microscopy of bone marrow in rabbit. Scand J Clin Lab Invest 1959;11(S38):1–82.
4. Mavrogenis AF, Dimitriou R, Parvizi J, et al. Biology of implant osseointegration. J Musculoskelet Neuronal Interact 2009;9(2):61–71.
5. Branemark PI, Adell R, Albrektsson T, et al. Osseointegrated titanium fixtures in the treatment of edentulousness. Biomaterials 1983;4:25–8.
6. Eriksson AR, Albrektsson T. Temperature threshold levels for heat-induced bone tissue injury: a vital-microscopic study in the rabbit. J Prosthet Dent 1983;50(1): 101–7.
7. Wilson CH, Clegg RE, Leavesley DI, et al. Mediation of biomaterial-cell interactions by adsorbed proteins: a review. Tissue Eng 2005;11:1–18.
8. Bruder SP, Fink DJ, Caplan AI. Mesenchymal stem cells in bone development, bone repair, and skeletal regeneration therapy. J Cell Biochem 1994;56:283–94.
9. Neuss S, Schneider RK, Tietze L, et al. Secretion of fibrinolytic enzymes facilitates human mesenchymal stem cell invasion into fibrin clots. Cells Tissues Organs 2010;191:36–46.
10. Berglundh T, Abrahamsson I, Lang NP, et al. De novo alveolar bone formation adjacent to endosseous implants. Clin Oral Implants Res 2003;14:251–62.
11. Meyer U, Joos U, Mythili J, et al. Ultrastructural characterization of the implant/bone interface of immediately loaded dental implants. Biomaterials 2004;25: 1959–67.
12. Murai K, Takeshita F, Ayukawa Y, et al. Light and electron microscopic studies of bone-titanium interface in the tibiae of young and mature rat. J Biomed Mater Res 1996;30:523–33.
13. Lang NP, Salvi GE, Huynh-Ba S, et al. Early osseointegration to hydrophilic and hydrophobic implant surfaces in humans. Clin Oral Implants Res 2011;22: 349–56.

14. Mulari MT, Qu Q, Harkonen PI. Osteoblast-like cells complete osteoclastic bone reportion and form new mineralized bone matrix in vitro. Calcif Tissue Int 2003;75: 253–61.
15. Bragdon CR, Burke D, Lowenstein JD, et al. Differences in stiffness of the interface between a cementless porous implant and cancellous bone in vivo in dogs due to varying amounts of implant motion. J Arthroplasty 1996;11:945–51.
16. Thalji G, Cooper LF. Molecular assessment of osseointegration in vitro: a review of current literature. Int J Oral Maxillofac Implants 2014;29(2):e171–99.
17. Miron RJ, Bosshardt DD. OsteoMacs: key players around bone biomaterials. Biomaterials 2016;92:1–19.
18. Ribeiro FV, Cesar-Neto JB, Nociti FH, et al. Selective cyclooxygenase-2 inhibitor may impair bone healing around titanium implants in rats. J Periodontol 2006;77: 1731–5.
19. Gomes FIF, Aragao MGB, de Paulo Teixeira Pinto V, et al. Effects of nonsteroidal anti-inflammatory drugs on osseointegration: a review. J Oral Implantol 2015;41: 219–30.
20. Chang MK, Raggatt LJ, Alexander KA, et al. Osteal tissue macrophages are intercalated throughout human and mous bone lining tissues and regulate osteoblast function in vitro and in vivo. J Immunol 2008;181(2):1232–44.
21. Kobayashi K, Takahashi N, Jimi E, et al. Tumor necrosis factor alpha stimulates osteoclast differentiation by a mechanism independent of ODF/RANKL-RANK interaction. J Exp Med 2000;191:275–86.
22. Assoian RK, Fleurdelys BE, Stevenson HC, et al. Expression and secretion of type beta transforming growth factor by activated human macrophages. Proc Natl Acad Sci U S A 1987;84:6020–4.
23. Itoh K, Udagawa N, Kobayashi K, et al. Lipopolysaccharide promotes the survival of osteoblasts via Toll-like receptor 4, but cytokine production of osteoclasts in response to lipopolysaccharide is different from that of macrophages. J Immunol 2003;170:3688–95.
24. Jimi E, Nakamura I, Duong LT, et al. Interleukin 1 induces multinucleation and bone-resorbing activity of osteoclasts in the absence of osteoblasts/stromal cells. Exp Cell Res 1999;247:84–93.
25. Takahashi F, Takahashi K, Shimizu K, et al. Osteopontin is strongly expressed by alveolar macrophages in the lungs of acute respiratory distress syndrome. Lung 2004;182:173–85.
26. Kreutz M, Andreesen R, Krause SW, et al. 1,25-dihydroxyvitamin D3 production and vitamin D3 receptor expression are developmentally regulated during differentiation of human monocytes into macrophages. Blood 1993;82:1300–7.
27. Champagne CM, Takebe J, Offenbacher S, et al. Macrophage cells lines produce osteoinducive signals that include bone morphogenic protein-2. Bone 2002;30: 26–31.
28. Vasconcelos DP, Costa M, Amaral IF, et al. Modulation of the inflammatory response to chitosan through M2 macrophage polarization using pro-resolution mediators. Biomaterials 2015;37:116–23.
29. Winkler IG, Sims NA, Pettit AR, et al. Bone marrow macrophages maintain hematopoietic stem cell (HSC) niches and their depletion mobilizes HSCs. Blood 2010;116:4815–28.
30. Van Wesenbeeck L, Odgren PR, MacKay CA, et al. The osteopetrotic mutation toothless (tl) is a loss-of-function frameshift mutation in the rat Csf1 gene: evidence of a crucial role of CSF-1 in osteoclastogenesis and endochondral ossification. Proc Natl Acad Sci U S A 2002;99:14303–8.

31. Kong YY, Yoshida H, Sarosi I, et al. OPGL is a key regulator os osteoclastogenesis, lymphocyte development and lymph node organogenesis. Nature 1999; 397:315–23.

32. Duong LT, Lakkakorpi P, Nakamura I, et al. Integrins and signaling in osteoclast function. Matrix Biol 2000;19:97–105.

33. Brodbeck WG, Anderson JM. Giant cell formation and function. Curr Opin Hematol 2009;16:53–7.

34. Pettit AR, Chang MK, Hume DA, et al. Osteal macrophages: a new twist on coupling during bone dynamics. Bone 2008;43:976–82.

35. Milleret V, Tugulu S, Schlottig F, et al. Alkali treatment of microrough titanium surfaces affects macrophage/monocyte adhesion, platelet activation and architecture of blood clot formation. Eur Cell Mater 2011;21:430–44.

36. Brinkmann J, Hefti T, Schlottig F. Response of osteoclasts to titanium surfaces with increasing surface roughness: an in vitro study. Biointerphases 2012;7:34.

37. Takebe J, Champagne CM, Offenbacher S, et al. Titanium surface topography alters cell shape and modules bone morphogenetic protein 2 expression in the J774A.1 macrophage cell line. J Biomed Mater Res 2003;64:207–16.

38. Barth KA, Waterfield JD, Brunette DM. The effect of surface roughness on RAW264.7 macrophage phenotype. J Biomed Mater Res 2013;101:2679–88.

39. Makihira S, Mine Y, Kosaka E, et al. Titanium surface roughness accelerates RANKL-dependent differentiation in the osteoclast precursor cell line, RAW264.7. Dent Mater J 2007;26:739–45.

40. Hong DGK, Oh J. Recent advances in dental implants. Maxillofac Plast Reconstr Surg 2017;39:33–42.

41. Wennerberg A, Albrektsson T. Effects of titanium surface topography on bone integration: a systematic review. Clin Oral Implants Res 2009;20(S4):172–84.

42. Larsson A, Wigren S, Andersson M, et al. Histologic evaluation of soft tissue integration of experimental abutments for bone anchored hearing implants using surgery without soft tissue reduction. Otol Neurotol 2012;33:1445–51.

43. Hawley K, Haberkamp TJ. Osseointegrated hearing implant surgery: outcomes using a minimal soft tissue removal technique. Otolaryngol Head Neck Surg 2013;149:653–7.

44. Hultcrantz M. Outcome of the bone-anchored hearing aid procedure without skin thinning: a prospective clinical trial. Otol Neurotol 2011;32:1134–9.

45. Husseman J, Szudek J, Monksfield P, et al. Simplified bone-anchored hearing aid insertion using a linear incision without soft tissue reduction. J Laryngol Otol 2013;127:S33–8.

46. Wilkie MD, Chakravarthy KM, Mamais C, et al. Osseointegrated hearing implant surgery using a novel hydroxyapatite-coated concave abutment design. Otolaryngol Head Neck Surg 2014;151(6):1014–9.

47. Rocci M, Rocci A, Martignoni M, et al. Comparing the TiOblast and Osseospeed surfaces: histomorphometric and histological analysis in humans. Oral Implantol (Rome) 2008;1:34–42.

48. Foghsgaard S, Caye-Thomasen P. A new wide-diameter bone-anchored hearing implant: prospective 1-year data on complications, implant stability, and survival. Otol Neurotol 2014;35(7):1238–41.

49. Shah FA, Johansson ML, Omar O, et al. Laser-modified surface enhances osseointegration and biomechanical anchorage of commercially pure titanium implants for bone-anchored hearing systems. PLoS One 2016;11(6):1–24.

50. Taghavi H, Hakansson B, Eeg-Olofsson M, et al. A vibration investigation of a flat surface contact to skull bone for direct bone conduction transmission in sheep skulls in vivo. Otol Neurotol 2013;34:690–8.
51. Jenny G, Jauernik J, Bierbaum S, et al. A systematic review and meta-analysis on the influence of biological implant surface coatings on periimplant bone formation. J Biomed Mater Res 2016;104:2898–910.
52. Dun VA, Faber HT, de Wolf MT, et al. Assessment of more than 1000 implanted percutaneous bone conduct devices: skin reactions and implant survival. Otol Neurotol 2012;33:192–8.
53. Kiringoda R, Lustig LR. A meta-analysis of the complications associated with osseointegrated hearing aids. Otol Neurotol 2013;34(5):790–4.
54. Wong MM, Rao LG, Ly H, et al. In vitro study of osteoblastic cells from patients with idiopathic osteoporosis and comparison with cells from non-osteoporotic controls. Osteoporos Int 1994;4:21–31.
55. Fini M, Giavaresi G, Torricelli P, et al. Biocompatibility and osseointegration in osteoporotic bone. J Bone Joint Surg Br 2001;83:139–43.
56. Chacon GE, Stine EA, Larsen PET, et al. Effect of alendronate on endosseous implant integration: an in vivo study in rabbits. J Oral Maxillofac Surg 2006;64:1005–9.
57. Eberhardt C, Habermann B, Mueller S, et al. The bisphosphonate ibandronate accelerates osseointegration of hydroxyapatite-coated cementless implants in an animal model. J Orthop Sci 2007;12:61–6.
58. Ayukawa Y, Okamura A, Koyano K. Sivastatin promotes osteogenesis around titanium implants. Clin Oral Implants Res 2004;15:346–50.
59. Sumner DR, Turner TM, Pierson RH, et al. Effects of radiation on fixation of non-cemented porous-coated implants in a canine model. J Bone Joint Surg Am 1990;72:1527–33.
60. Bolind P, Johannson CB, Johansson P, et al. Retrieved implants from irradiated sites in humans: a histologic/histomorphometric investigation of oral and craniofacial implants. Clin Implant Dent Relat Res 2006;8:142–50.

Osseointegrated Auditory Devices

Bone-Anchored Hearing Aid and PONTO

Soha N. Ghossaini, MD[a],*, Pamela C. Roehm, MD, PhD[b]

KEYWORDS

- Osseointegrated auditory device • Osseointegrated auditory implant • BAHA
- Ponto • Single-sided deafness • Conductive hearing loss • Mixed hearing loss

KEY POINTS

- Osseointegrated auditory devices (OADs) allow direct coupling of a bone-conduction processor to the calvarium.
- Low power is needed to conduct sound to the target cochlea, allowing treatment of patients with higher (worse) bone-conduction thresholds.
- Indications that a patient would be a good candidate for OADs include unilateral or bilateral conductive and mixed hearing loss and single-sided deafness.
- Modifications in surgical techniques and design of OADs have resulted in reducing soft tissue complications.

INTRODUCTION

Osseointegrated auditory devices (OADs) incorporate a titanium prosthesis that is implanted into the calvarium.[1] Once osseointegration occurs (1–3 months), an external receiver/processor can be attached, allowing bone conduction of sound directly to the target cochlea (**Fig. 1**). Processor attachment can be achieved either by direct attachment via a percutaneous abutment ("connect" systems) or via transcutaneous magnetic attraction; please see Dr C.Y. Joseph Chang's article, "Ossicle Coupling Active Implantable Auditory Devices: Magnetic Driven System," in this issue for further information. Due to direct conduction through OADs, less power is required to transmit sound than for traditional bone-conduction hearing aids.[2] The first OAD was developed in the 1970s. As OAD technology has advanced (**Table 1**), indications have expanded (**Box 1**).[3] Although there are some differences between the 2 currently approved devices being discussed in this article, the overall assessment, surgical technique, and trouble-shooting for potential complications is similar. Therefore, the following applies to both the bone-anchored hearing aid (BAHA) and PONTO OAD systems.

---

[a] Otology-Neurotology, Ear Nose and Throat Associates of New York, 107-21 Queens Boulevard, Forest Hills, NY 11375, USA; [b] Department of Otolaryngology—Head and Neck Surgery, Temple University School of Medicine, 3509 North Broad Street, Suite 300, Philadelphia, PA 19140, USA
* Corresponding author. 27-18 Hoyt Avenue South, Apartment 8B, Astoria, NY 11102.
E-mail address: sghossaini@gmail.com

Otolaryngol Clin N Am 52 (2019) 243–251
https://doi.org/10.1016/j.otc.2018.11.005
0030-6665/19/© 2018 Elsevier Inc. All rights reserved.

oto.theclinics.com

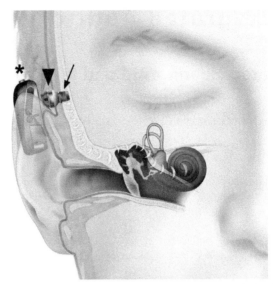

Fig. 1. Components of OADs. The primary components of OADs include the implant (*arrow*) and abutment (*arrowhead*). After osseointegration, a bone-conduction processor is attached to the abutment (*asterisk*). (With permission by Cochlear Americas, Englewood, CO.)

AUDITORY INDICATIONS FOR OSSEOINTEGRATED AUDITORY DEVICES

OADs can be used to stimulate the ipsilateral cochlea in cases of unilateral or bilateral conductive hearing loss (CHL) (**Box 1**).[3] For mixed conductive and sensorineural

Table 1	
History of osseointegrated auditory devices	
1997	Initial implantation of percutaneous custom made OADs in Europe for CHL (Anders Tjellstrom)
1985	First bone-conduction sound processor (HC-100) becomes commercially available
1995	First miniaturized sound processor (BAHA 360) released
1996–1997	FDA approval of BAHA for patients >18 y old with unilateral CHL or MHL
1997	First superpower sound processor released (Cordelle)
1999	Snap coupling introduced for BAHA processor (Cordelle II)
1999	FDA approval of BAHA for patients >5 y old with unilateral CHL or MHL
2001	FDA approval of BAHA for bilateral implantation in patients >5 y old with CHL or MHL
2002	FDA approval of BAHA for SSD
2005	Ear level digital sound processor released (Divino)
2007	First head-worn power device released (Intenso)
2009	FDA approval of the PONTO (Oticon) for unilateral or bilateral CHL and MHL AND for SSD

Abbreviations: CHL, conductive hearing loss; FDA, Food and Drug Administration; MHL, mixed conductive and sensorineural hearing loss; OAD, osseointegrated auditory device; SSD, single-sided sensorineural deafness.

Box 1
Audiometric indications

- Conductive hearing loss or mixed conductive and sensorineural hearing loss with bone-conduction thresholds ≤65 dB on the affected side
- Single-sided sensorineural deafness (SSD) with normal thresholds on the unaffected side
- SSD with decreased hearing thresholds less than 40 to 50 dB on the unaffected side

---

hearing losses (MHL), OADs can be used to stimulate either the ipsilateral or contralateral cochlea depending on the degree of ipsilateral sensorineural loss.[4] In addition, OADs can be used to treat single-sided sensorineural deafness (SSD) through conduction to the contralateral cochlea.[3,5] Current processors can effectively amplify to overcome ≤65 dB ipsilateral bone-conduction threshold (**Table 2**).

OSSEOINTEGRATED AUDITORY DEVICE MEDICAL INDICATIONS

OADs are particularly useful for patients who cannot be remediated using conventional hearing aids (CHAs) because of a variety of medical conditions. These include patients with absent external auditory canals due to congenital or acquired aural atresia or following temporal bone resection, particularly those who cannot tolerate a headband bone-conduction aid or who have a sensorineural component to the hearing loss in the target cochlea. Often, patients with infections (chronic suppurative otitis media or recurrent otitis externa) or other medical conditions that are worsened by CHA use can benefit from OADs. Patients with benign external auditory canal tumors (exostoses and osteoma) or with large meatoplasties who cannot be fitted comfortably with CHAs can successfully wear OADs. Finally, OADs can be useful for patients who cannot tolerate the occlusion effect of larger earmolds.[3]

EVALUATION

Preoperative auditory evaluation includes an audiogram and trial of an OAD processor attached via a bone-conduction headband; please see Maja Svrakic and Andrea Vambutas' article, "Medical and Audiological Indications for Implantable Auditory

---

Table 2
Processor amplification

Type	Variety of Loss	Bone-Conduction Threshold in the Target Cochlea
Conventional	CHL or MHL	≤45 dB HL
	SSD	0–20 dB HL
Power	CHL or MHL	≤55 dB
	SSD	0–30 dB, strong transcranial attenuation
Superpower	CHL or MHL	≤65 dB
	SSD	≤40–50 dB

Abbreviations: CHL, conductive hearing loss; HL, hearing loss; MHL, mixed conductive and sensorineural hearing loss; SSD, single-sided sensorineural deafness.

Devices," elsewhere in this issue for further information. Patients should be counseled that sound transmission via the trial will be lower in quality compared with transmission via the implanted device.[2] Temporal bone computed tomography without contrast should be used for patients who have previously had temporal bone resection or ipsilateral neurosurgical procedures and may be useful in preoperative planning for patients with craniofacial anomalies.[3]

CURRENT SURGICAL TECHNIQUE

Surgery can be performed in a number of settings (office, outpatient surgicenter, or operating room), depending on anesthesia requirements. Local anesthesia may be sufficient for the procedure for adults, but often light sedation is required. For younger children or adults with a language barrier, general anesthesia may be required.[3]

The incision is marked on the scalp and is typically linear and vertical, although other variants have been reported (**Fig. 2**).[6] The incision is typically 2 to 3 cm in length and is positioned 5.0 to 5.5 cm posterior to the pinna along the hairline, 30° superior to the superior aspect of the tragus or external auditory canal meatus. The implant site is marked (1 cm posterior to or within the incision line). The position of the implant can be adjusted for use of eyeglasses and headwear. The surgical site is sterilely prepped. Before injection of local anesthetic, a sterile needle is inserted to check scalp thickness to determine appropriate abutment length, which is 2 to 3 mm longer than the measured thickness.

The skin incision is carried down to the periosteum. The central periosteum over the planned implant site is incised in a cruciate pattern and elevated. The implant drill is used to make a 3-mm-deep well, and, if bone is palpated deep to that, a 4-mm implant drill is used to extend that well medially by 1 mm. An appropriately deep (3 or 4 mm) countersink well is also drilled. All of this bony removal is performed using high-speed drilling and copious irrigation.

For single-stage implantation, the implant and abutment are secured using the drill at lower torque, and irrigation after the first 2 turns to avoid heat to the area, as explained in Jennifer Wing Yee Lee and Manohar Lal Bance's article, "Physiology of Osseointegration," elsewhere in this issue. The abutment is brought out through the scalp either in the incision or via a separate dermal punch skin excision. The incision line is closed, and a pressure dressing is applied.

Two-staged surgeries are indicated for younger children, and patients whose cranial bone thickness is <3 mm or whose cranium has been irradiated.[3,7–9] For these

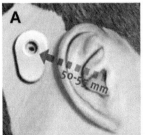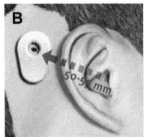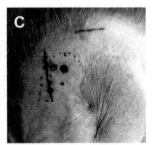

Fig. 2. Determining site of OAD implantation. (*A*) The implant site is marked 50 to 55 mm from the center of the ear canal. (*B*) An incision is marked anterior to the implant site. (*C*) OAD site marking after total auriculectomy, lateral temporal bone resection, and free flap. (*Courtesy of* Oticon Medical, Vallauris, France, with permission.)

patients, the implant is secured into the well to the appropriate depth available. A cover screw, which prevents ingrowth of soft tissue, is placed into the implant. The second stage is performed 3 to 6 months afterward. At that time, the skin over the implant is incised using a 5-mm biopsy punch. The cover screw is removed. The abutment is attached to the implant and tightened to 25 Ncm.

Simultaneous placement of a back-up or "sleeper" implant can be performed during either single-stage or 2-staged surgeries.[7] Backups are placed within ≥10 mm of the primary implant and covered with a cover screw (**Box 2**).

Newer techniques, including single-stage techniques using a large biopsy punch to make the only skin incision have been described. These techniques are promising for the future and may supplant the linear incision technique (**Fig. 3**).[10,11]

COMPLICATIONS

The most common complications following OAD placement involve the soft tissues around the abutment (**Box 3**). Soft tissue complications have decreased in frequency following the widespread use of soft tissue–sparing techniques and use of longer abutments. In a series of 223 ears, soft tissue complications occurred in 17.5% of patients, 4.5% requiring surgical revision.[12] Soft tissue complications are more common following head and neck irradiation.[9] Treatment for infectious complications includes topical or oral antibiotics and excision of granulation tissue. Rarely, a bacterially contaminated abutment will require removal to control infection. Abutment overgrowth by skin or granulation tissue can be treated with revision and placement of a longer abutment combined with control of infection. Keloid formation can be treated with steroid injection and compression, and excision as needed[12] (**Fig. 4**).

Failure of osseointegration or delayed osseous disintegration occurs in 1.3% to 26.0% of patients.[12–16] Risk factors include trauma, incomplete insertion of the implant, and younger patient age at implantation.[12,17] Infectious skin complications may lead to osseous disintegration.[12] Treatment includes removal with implantation at another site.

HEARING OUTCOMES

OADs can yield excellent hearing outcomes in both unilateral and bilateral CHL.[3] Four-frequency (500, 1000, 2000, 4000 Hz) air conduction averages improve from 60.8 unaided to 30.6 dB hearing loss (HL) with percutaneous OADs.[3,12,18] Patient satisfaction in this group of patients is high, with most wearing the OAD daily and reporting significant improvements in quality of life.[1,19,20]

Due to transcranial attenuation of bone conduction (−5 dB to 20 dB HL), patients with bilateral CHL can benefit from bilateral OADs.[21] Systematic review of patients with bilateral CHL and bilateral OAD placements demonstrated improvement of hearing in quiet (pure tone average ≥15 dB, speech reception 4.0–5.4 dB, and word recognition ≥5.5% compared with unilateral OAD).[22] In noise, hearing

---

Box 2
Indications for sleeper implantation

- Calvarial bone thickness <3 to 4 mm
- Younger patient age (<10 years)
- Surgeon preference

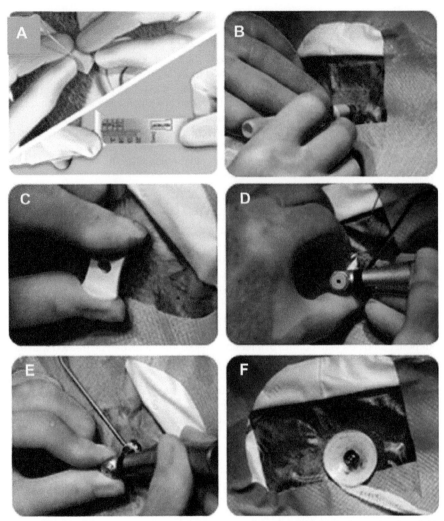

Fig. 3. Minimally invasive percutaneous OAD procedure. (*A*) Position is determined and skin thickness measured. (*B*) Incision of skin and soft tissues. (*C*) A protective canula protects surrounding tissues. (*D*) The well is drilled. (*E*) Implant insertion. (*F*) A healing cap is placed. (*Courtesy of* Oticon Medical, Vallauris, France; with permission.)

Box 3
Soft tissue complications of osseointegrated auditory device placement

- Erythema and tenderness of skin around abutment
- Granulation tissue
- Cellulitis
- Abscess
- Skin overgrowth of abutment
- Hypertrophic scars and keloids

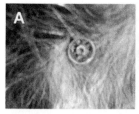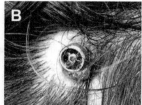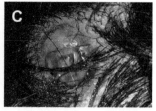

Fig. 4. Infectious complications of OADs. Erythema around the abutment (*A*), granulation tissue (*B*), soft tissue overgrowth (*C*).

outcomes also improved (speech reception $\geq$3.1 dB, word recognition $\geq$14%). Localization of sound improved from chance levels to near-normal when patients were tested in the bilateral state.[22] Patient-based subjective outcomes and satisfaction are high with bilateral OADs.[22] Ninety percent of patients wore both processors 7 days a week, with the other 10% of users wearing processors at least 5 to 6 days per week[23]

For patients with MHL and bone thresholds $\leq$60 to 65 dB HL, hearing outcomes and patient satisfaction results similar to those seen for patients with CHL can be anticipated with use of an appropriately powered processor.[3,4,19]

With SSD and normal hearing in the contralateral ear, patients can anticipate improvement in speech discrimination in noise, with results varying from -3.8 to -4.8 dB signal-to-noise ratio depending on noise location.[5] Although some studies have found improved sound location, typically sound localization is not significantly better than in the unaided condition with SSD and an OAD.[5] Nonetheless, all studies have demonstrated significant improvement in quality of life for patients with SSD with an OAD.

Patients with SSD and contralateral sensorineural HL can anticipate improvement as long as the processor is sufficiently powered.[3] Schwartz and colleagues[24] demonstrated that improvement in quality of life was the same in these nontraditional candidates compared with patients with SSD and normal contralateral hearing. Due to the variability of hearing in these patients, measurements of hearing improvement are difficult to generalize. Nontraditional patients with SSD did slightly worse on functional measures of hearing, including hearing in noise, compared with more typical patients with SSD with an OAD. Sound localization was equally poor in nontraditional candidates compared with SSD and normal contralateral hearing (62.7 vs 53.3). These patients must be counseled that their OAD may become less effective over time, as HL in the better-hearing ear progresses.[24]

SUMMARY

OADs can treat a wide variety of HLs, including unilateral and bilateral CHL, unilateral and bilateral MHL, and SSD. New surgical techniques have shortened operative times and decreased complications. Limitations to OADs need to be understood by patients before implantation.

REFERENCES

1. Tjellström A, Lindström J, Hallén O, et al. Osseointegrated titanium implants in the temporal bone. A clinical study on bone-anchored hearing aids. Am J Otol 1981; 2(4):304–10.

2. Verstraeten N, Zarowski AJ, Somers T, et al. Comparison of the audiologic results obtained with the bone-anchored hearing aid attached to the headband, the test-band, and to the "snap" abutment. Otol Neurotol 2009;30(1):70–5.

3. Spitzer JB, Ghossaini SN, Wazen JJ. Evolving applications in the use of bone-anchored hearing aids. Am J Audiol 2002;11(2):96–103.

4. Wazen JJ, Caruso M, Tjellström A. Long-term results with the titanium bone-anchored hearing aid: the U.S. experience. Am J Otol 1998;19(6):737–41.

5. Kim G, Ju HM, Lee SH, et al. Efficacy of bone-anchored hearing aids in single-sided deafness: a systematic review. Otol Neurotol 2017;38(4):473–83.

6. Hultcrantz M, Lanis A. A five-year follow-up on the osseointegration of bone-anchored hearing device implantation without tissue reduction. Otol Neurotol 2014;35(8):1480–5.

7. Davids T, Gordon KA, Clutton D, et al. Bone-anchored hearing aids in infants and children younger than 5 years. Arch Otolaryngol Head Neck Surg 2007;133(1): 51–5.

8. Soo G, Tong MC, Tsang WS, et al. The BAHA hearing system for hearing-impaired postirradiated nasopharyngeal cancer patients: a new indication. Otol Neurotol 2009;30(4):496–501.

9. Wilkie MD, Lightbody KA, Salamat AA, et al. Stability and survival of bone-anchored hearing aid implant systems in post-irradiated patients. Eur Arch Oto-rhinolaryngol 2015;272(6):1371–6.

10. Gordon SA, Coelho DH. Minimally invasive surgery for osseointegrated auditory implants: a comparison of linear versus punch techniques. Otolaryngol Head Neck Surg 2015;152(6):1089–93.

11. Calon TGA, van Hoof M, van den Berge H, et al. Minimally Invasive Ponto surgery compared to the linear incision technique without soft tissue reduction for bone conduction hearing implants: study protocol for a randomized controlled trial. Trials 2016;17(1):540.

12. Wazen JJ, Young DL, Farrugia MC, et al. Successes and complications of the BAHA system. Otol Neurotol 2008;29(8):115–9.

13. Reyes RA, Tjellström A, Granstrom G. Evaluation of implant losses and skin reactions around extraoral bone-anchored implants, a 0- to 8-year follow-up. Otolaryngol Head Neck Surg 2000;122(2):272–6.

14. House JW, Kutz JW. Bone-anchored hearing aids: incidence and management of postoperative complications. Otol Neurotol 2007;28(2):213–7.

15. Proops DW. The Birmingham bone anchored hearing aid programme: surgical methods and complications. J Laryngol Otol Suppl 1996;21:7–12.

16. Lloyd S, Almeyda J, Sirimanna KS, et al. Updated surgical experience with bone-anchored hearing aids in children. J Laryngol Otol 2007;121(9):826–31.

17. Zeitoun H, De R, Thompson SD, et al. Osseointegrated implants in the management of childhood ear abnormalities: with particular emphasis on complications. J Laryngol Otol 2002;116(2):87–91.

18. Powell HRF, Rolfe AM, Birman CS. A comparative study of audiologic outcomes for two transcutaneous bone-anchored hearing devices. Otol Neurotol 2015; 36(9):1525–31.

19. Mylanus EAM, Snik AFM, Jorritsma FF, et al. Audiologic results for the bone-anchored hearing aid HC220. Ear Hear 1994;15(1):87–92.

20. Banga R, Doshi J, Child A, et al. Bone-anchored hearing devices in children with unilateral conductive hearing loss: a patient-carer perspective. Ann Otol Rhinol Laryngol 2013;122(9):582–7.

21. Nolan M, Lyon DJ. Transcranial attenuation in bone conduction audiometry. J Laryngol Otol 1981;95(6):597–608.
22. Janssen RM, Hong P, Chadha NK. Bilateral bone-anchored hearing aids for bilateral permanent conductive hearing loss: a systematic review. Otolaryngol Head Neck Surg 2012;147(3):412–22.
23. Dun CAJ, de Wolf MJF, Mylanus EAM, et al. Bilateral bone-anchored hearing aid application in children: the Nijmegen experience from 1996-2008. Otol Neurotol 2010;31(4):615–23.
24. Schwartz SR, Kobylk D. Outcomes of bone anchored hearing aids (BAHA) for single sided deafness in nontraditional candidates. Otol Neurotol 2016;37(10): 1608–13.

Osseointegrated Auditory Devices—Transcutaneous

Sophono and Baha Attract

Darius Kohan, MD[a],*, Soha N. Ghossaini, MD[b]

KEYWORDS

- Transcutaneous • Bone anchored • Osseointegrated • Sophono • Baha Attract

KEY POINTS

- Transcutaneous bone-anchored auditory implants are safe, effective, and cosmetically acceptable, with low complication rates.
- Transcutaneous implants outcome as performed in both children and adults, provide up to 40dB gain, usually superior to Softband attached auditory processors.
- Percutaneous auditory implants generally provide 5 to 7 dB superior gain versus transcutaneous devices owing to direct coupling of processor to fixture/implant.
- Transcutaneous implantable auditory devices are MRI compatible; however, the Baha Attract has an 11-cm shadow versus 5 cm for the Sophono.

INTRODUCTION

Percutaneous osseointegrated bone conduction implants, as noted by Soha N. Ghossaini and Pamela C. Roehm's article, "Osseointegrated Auditory Devices: BAHA and PONTO," in this issue, are well-documented to be a very effective modality for auditory rehabilitation in appropriate clinical settings. The main complications of percutaneous devices are related to the inflammatory interaction between the abutment and surrounding skin. In earlier studies, up to 30% of these patients had skin overgrowth or infections at the abutment site. Many modifications and improvements have occurred over time to ameliorate this problem; however, the cosmetic and psychological issue of a "pin sticking out of one's head" has not gone away. Transcutaneous osseointegrated devices were developed to address these issues.[1] The Sophono system (Sophono, Inc, Boulder, CO) was the first to develop this technology, soon to be followed by the Baha Attract (Cochlear Ltd, Sydney, Australia). The acceptable medical

Disclosure Statement: D. Kohan: Medtronics- Principal investigator of Clinical trial comparing Osseointegrated bone conduction devices 2014/15. S. Ghossaini: none.
[a] Otolaryngology NYU School of Medicine, Northwell Health System, 863 Park Avenue, Suite1E, New York, NY 10075, USA; [b] Otology- Neurotology, Ear Nose and Throat Associates of New York, 35-30 Francis Lewis Boulevard, Auburndale, NY 11358, USA
* Corresponding author.
E-mail address: earmaven@aol.com

oto.theclinics.com

diagnoses by insurance carriers in the United States are the same regardless if osseointegrated devices are transcutaneous or percutaneous (**Box 1**). The US Food and Drug Administration-approved indications for the Sophono and Baha Attract are the same (**Box 2**).

SOPHONO: MAGNETIC BONE CONDUCTION HEARING SYSTEM

The Sophono system consists of a titanium encased magnetic implant, a magnetic spacer baseplate, and the Alpha 2 MPO sound processor. The magnetic implant is the smallest on the market and lies completely under the skin. It consists of 2 magnets hermetically sealed in a titanium case (**Fig. 1**).

Percutaneous devices transmit sound energy directly into bone via a sound processor that is coupled to an implanted abutment screw. In this transcutaneous device, the sound vibrations are transmitted via a baseplate to the skin, the implant magnet, and the 5 osseointegrated maxillofacial screws securing the implant to bone, thus allowing for bone conduction to the cochlea bilaterally. The size of the baseplate in contact with the skin is important for maximum transfer of power to the bone. Transcutaneous energy transfer technology may eliminate up to 20 dB of energy reflection on skin typically associated with percutaneous systems. The maximum acoustic gain is 45 dB. The more direct energy transfer from processor to bone in percutaneous devices allows for a 5- to 7-dB theoretic gain advantage versus transcutaneous transmission (**Figs. 2** and **3**).[1] The Sophono is cleared by the US Food and Drug Administration for MRI conditional up to 3 T. The Sophono implant magnet produces a 5-cm shadow versus an 11-cm shadow by the Baha Attract magnet, and in both systems magnet removal is not required.

Surgical Technique

The procedure may be performed under general anesthesia or monitored sedation and should take about 30 to 45 minutes. A sterile template is provided with the implant to facilitate flap design (**Fig. 4**).

Box 1
Acceptable medical diagnoses for osseointegrated implants (Baha, Ponto, SOPHONO): _International Classification of Disease_ codes

Anomalies
  744.0: Anomalies of ear causing hearing impairment
  744.23: Microtia
  380.50: Acquired stenosis EAC

Infections:
  380.02: Chronic perichondritis of pinna
  380.14-6: Chronic otitis externa
  380.53: Acquired stenosis EAC
  381.1-4: Chronic serous otitis
  382.0-01: Acute otitis media
  385.3: Cholesteatoma

Hearing loss:
  389.01-03 Conductive hearing loss
  387 Otosclerosis
  389.21-22: Mixed hearing loss
  389.13: Single-sided deafness

Abbreviation: EAC, external auditory canal.

Courtesy of Andrea Vambutas, MD, Hempstead, NY.

Box 2
FDA-approved indications for transcutaneous osseointegrated devices

- Conductive hearing loss
- Mixed hearing loss
- SSD
- Age 5 to adult (implanted); all ages (headband/softband)
- $\leq$45 dB bone conduction thresholds for indicated ear
- $\leq$20 dB bone conduction thresholds in the better hearing ear (SSD)

Abbreviations: FDA, US Food and Drug Administration; SSD, single-sided deafness.

A semicircular incision is carried to the periosteum, which is elevated with the skin flap. A template of the implant magnet is used to drill down 2 wells (2 mm deep) to accommodate the implant, which must be secured in appropriate orientation with 5 maxillofacial screws of 3/4 mm length (**Fig. 5**).

An alternative that avoids bone drilling the 2 wells is to flip the magnet (sunny side up; **Fig. 6**). The skin overlying magnet should be between 4 and 8 mm thick. The incision is closed in layers. The device is usually activated at 6 weeks when the edema of the skin flap dissipated; however, if well-healed it may be activated as early as 3 weeks. The baseplate magnet comes in many different strengths to allow good coupling of the processor without skin irritation.

Complications

Complications with transcutaneous devices are exceedingly rare and related to the skin thickness over the implant. If too thin, patients report heat and discomfort wearing processor and skin may breakdown exposing implant. This complication may be addressed by decreasing the magnet strength of the baseplate. If the skin flap is too thick and the processor is not well-attached to implant site, one can increase the baseplate magnet strength to compensate. Revision surgery may also be indicated to address patient dissatisfaction, worsening hearing, and device obsolescence, as well as provide new and improved technology.

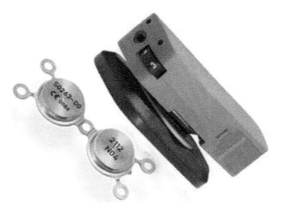

Fig. 1. Sophono implant magnet, baseplate magnet, and Alpha 2 MPO processor. (*Courtesy of* Medtronic, Minneapolis, MN; with permission.)

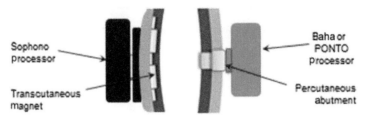

Fig. 2. Differences between transcutaneous and percutaneous transfer of sound vibration energy. Both put comparable energy into the temporal bone. The approaches differ, but both get to the same place. (*Courtesy of* Medtronic, Minneapolis, MN; with permission.)

Data on pediatric transcutaneous implantable auditory devices are limited. Denoyelle and colleagues[2] in a prospective study in 15 children with atresia implanted with the Sophono had no complications at all. Marsell and colleagues[3] in a study on 6 children with the Sophono had 1 child with mild pain with prolonged use of device with superficial ulceration that healed by lowering the baseplate magnet strength and with local skin care.

Results

O'Niel[4] studied the Sophono system in a pediatric population and concluded it was equally effective to the other Bone conduction (BC) systems. Other publications also found equivalent results among transcutaneous systems. A few studies compared the different transcutaneous systems. In 2016 a study limited to 26 patients comparing the Baha and Sophono systems, Kohan et al[5] (pending publication) concluded the percutaneous Baha with a #5 processor provided the best gain in pure tone average, followed by the Sophono with the Alpha 2 MPO processor, and the Baha Attract with a #5 processor (Kohan D, et al. Comparing hearing outcomes in osseointegrated implantable auditory devices," poster presented at, COSM)[5] (**Table 1**). The 6-dB pure tone average additional gain noted in the percutaneous relative to the best transcutaneous outcome is to be expected owing to the direct transmission of vibratory energy with an abutment versus a transcutaneous device.[6–8] The gain at high frequencies drops off for all devices (**Fig. 7**). The Sophono Alpha 2 MPO had the greatest percentage of gain achieved in pure tone average 4. Percutaneous Baha devices had a greater percentage of gain achieved compared with their transcutaneous counterparts (**Fig. 8**).

THE BAHA ATTRACT OSSEOINTEGRATED SYSTEM

The Baha Attract System is a new, passive, transcutaneous auditory osseointegrated device that was introduced into the market in 2013 in an attempt to overcome some of

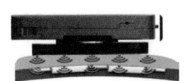
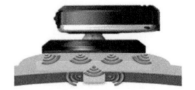

Fig. 3. The difference in the 2 transcutaneous systems. The Sophono, on the left, uses a proprietary transcutaneous energy transfer technology, whereas the Baha Attract (*right*) transmits energy to a baseplate that is attached to a single osseointegrated screw. (*Courtesy of* Medtronic, Minneapolis, MN; with permission.)

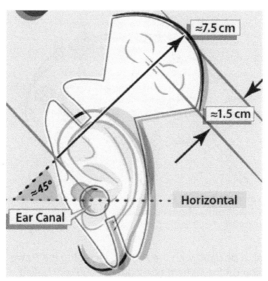

Fig. 4. SOPHONO surgical technique template localizes the incision site, length, and implant position. (*Courtesy of* Medtronic, Minneapolis, MN; with permission.)

the skin complications and aesthetic concerns of its percutaneous counterpart. It involves an osseointegrated titanium implant that is attached to an internal magnet. The external sound processor fits on a sound processor magnet that connects to the internal magnet transcutaneously. Theoretically, the intervening skin layer may result in less efficient sound transmission.[9,10] This limitation can, however, be overcome to a certain extent by the powerful sound processor in an auditory osseointegrated device as shown by the positive results in the literature.[11]

The indications for Baha Attract are the same as for the percutaneous Baha. However, per manufacturer recommendation, patients with single-sided deafness with large transcranial attenuation or hearing loss in the better hearing ear are better served with the Baha Connect. The same Baha processors available for the Connect version

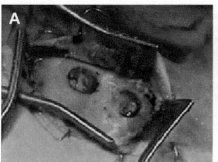
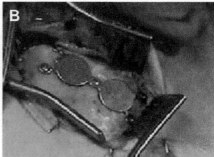

Fig. 5. Sophono surgical technique: operative photos. (*A*) Bone wells drilled into the bone using a the male template provided in the implant kit. (*B*) Implant magnet in place. Five 4-mm titanium screws are used for implant fixation. (*Courtesy of* Medtronic, Minneapolis, MN; with permission.)

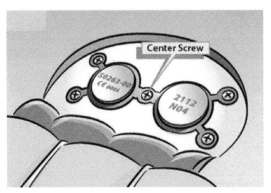

Fig. 6. Minimally invasive technique (sunny side up). No drilling is required; the device is flipped. (*Courtesy of* Medtronic, Minneapolis, MN; with permission.)

of the device may also be used with the Attract, including the Power and Superpower processor, depending on the patients presurgical auditory deficit.

Surgical Technique

Surgery can be performed under local or general anesthesia.[12,13] The implant site is identified using the template for Baha Attract ensuring that the sound processor and its magnet are not touching the pinna. This placement usually corresponds with a distance of 50 to 70 mm from the ear canal (**Fig. 9**). A C-shaped incision is marked on the scalp 15 mm away from the edge of the magnet (**Fig. 10**). The surgical site is prepared and sterilized. Before the injection of a local vasoconstrictive anesthetic, a sterile needle is inserted to check the scalp thickness. Soft tissue reduction is performed if the skin flap thickness is greater then 6 mm.

The skin incision is carried down to the periosteum and the flap is elevated. The implant magnet template is used to check for proper positioning of the implant magnet

Table 1
Audiometric gain observed among osseointegrated implantable auditory devices

	Baha Connect #4 Processor (dB)	Baha Connect #5 Processor (dB)	Baha Attract #4 Processor (dB)	Baha Attract #5 Processor (dB)	Sophono Alpha 2 Processor (dB)	Sophono Alpha 2 MPO Processor (dB)
PTA4 unaided implant ear	79	96	77	81	76	77
PTA4 unaided better ear (BC)	28	22	24	24	30	27
Max potential gain PTA4	51	74	53	57	46	50
Average gain	31	49	22	35	35	43
Average Res. ABG	20	25	31	22	11	7

Abbreviation: PTA4, pure tone average 4 (includes 4 frequencies: 500, 1000, 2000, 4000 Hz).
Courtesy of Darius Kohan, MD, New York, NY.

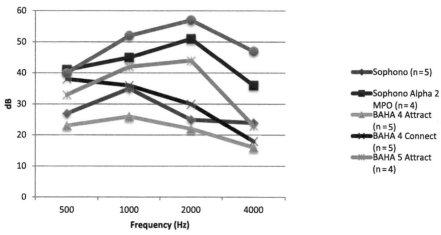

Fig. 7. Mean pure tone gain by device. All devices had a decrease in the mean gain at higher frequencies (4000 Hz). Of the transcutaneous devices, the Sophono Alpha 2 MPO had the least drop off. (*Courtesy of* Darius Kohan, MD, New York, NY; and Medtronic, Minneapolis, MN.)

against the skin flap and the underlying bone. The central periosteum over the planned implant site is incised in a cruciate pattern and elevated. The implant drill is used to make a 3-mm deep well, and, if bone is palpated deep to that, a 4-mm implant drill is used to extend that well medially by 1 mm. An appropriately deep (3 or 4 mm) countersink well is also drilled. All of this bony removal is performed using high-speed drilling and copious irrigation. For single-stage implantation, the implant is secured using

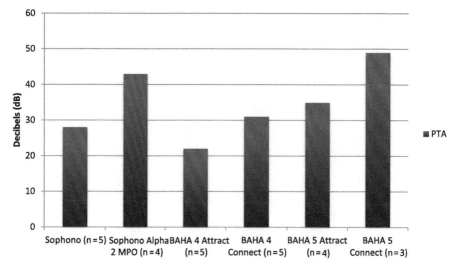

Fig. 8. Mean pure tone average 4 (PTA4) tone gain by device. The Sophono Alpha 2 MPO had the greatest percentage of gain achieved in PTA4. The percutaneous devices had greater percentage of gain achieved compared with their transcutaneous counterparts. (*Courtesy of* Darius Kohan, MD, New York, NY; and Medtronic, Minneapolis, MN.)

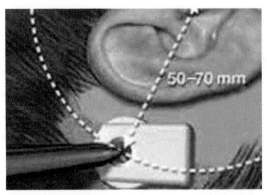

Fig. 9. The implant site usually corresponds with a distance of 50 to 70 mm from the ear canal. (*Courtesy of* Cochlear Limited, Sydney, Australia.)

the drill at lower torque, and irrigation after the first 2 turns to avoid excess heat to the area. Then the bone bed indicator is used to ensure that there is enough clearance for the implant magnet to sit flatly on the bone. If not, excess bone should be removed. Then the implant magnet is attached to the implant. The incision line is closed, and a pressure dressing is applied in Two-staged surgeries are indicated patients whose cranial bone thickness is less than 3 mm or whose cranium has been irradiated. For these patients, the implant is secured into the well to the appropriate depth available. A cover screw, which prevents the ingrowth of soft tissue, is placed into the implant. The second stage is performed 3 to 6 months later. At that time, the cover screw is removed and the implant magnet is placed.

It is also feasible to switch the Baha Connect to the Baha Attract for either cosmetic reasons or in patients with recurrent skin reactions from the percutaneous abutment.[14] In a similar fashion, A C-shaped incision is designed around the preexisting abutment making sure that it is 15 mm away from the edge of the magnet. The flap is elevated down to periosteum. The abutment is removed and the implant magnet is secured to the preexisting implant (**Fig. 11**). The flap is put back in position and adjacent tissue is undermined to allow for primary closure of the incision. The resultant skin defect from

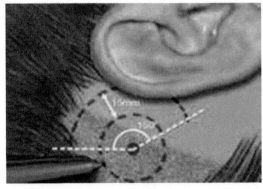

Fig. 10. A C-shaped incision is marked on the scalp 15 mm away from the edge of the magnet. (*Courtesy of* Cochlear Limited, Sydney, Australia.)

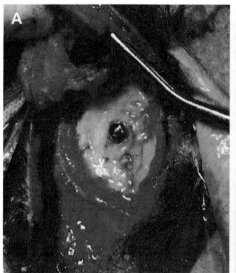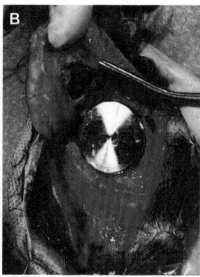

Fig. 11. Revision surgery from the Baha connect to attract. The Attract magnet is attached to original implant in (*B*) after abutment is removed as seen in (*A*). (*Courtesy of* Cochlear Limited, Sydney, Australia; and Sujana Chandrasekhar, MD, New York, NY.)

the site of the abutment is closed in a primary fashion if possible, or fascia or Alloderm may be used if there is a sizable skin defect.

Audiological results with the Baha Attract system revealed improved thresholds when compared with the unaided condition in most indications primarily in the speech frequency range. The threshold improvement was noted to be less above the 3000 Hz frequency. The audiological improvement postoperatively was comparable with the Baha band test results, indicating that Baha band test results are a good indicator of patient's benefit.[11]

In a recent multicenter study, Hougaard and colleagues,[12] looking at the benefits of Baha attract in 105 patients with conductive hearing loss/mixed hearing loss and single-sided deafness, it was found that free field audiometric testing scores improved mainly in the low and mid frequencies. Minimal improvements in the low and high frequencies were noticed in the single-sided deafness application. There was no significant improvement in hearing in noise for both the conductive hearing loss/missed hearing loss and the single-sided deafness group. Patients, however, reported subjective benefit with the device and small complication rate.

Dimitriadis and colleagues[13] in 2017 studied 105 Baha Attract patients with conductive hearing loss/mixed hearing loss and single-sided deafness. Of those who filled out the questionnaires, there was a significant improvement in patient-reported outcomes using the Glasgow Benefit Inventory and the Client Oriented Scale of Improvement for the adult population. A systematic review of the literature of Baha Attract patients in 2016 revealed satisfactory audiological results.[15] This review, however, looked for average improvement in audiological test scores of all patients with different types of hearing loss (conductive hearing loss/mixed hearing loss and single-sided deafness).

Iseri and colleagues[1] in 2015 compared the performance of 21 patients with conductive hearing loss with the percutaneous Baha with 16 patients with conductive hearing loss with the transcutaneous Baha Attract. It was noted that audiometric results for both groups were equivalent. No statistically significant differences were found in the frequency-specific hearing gains between the groups, but the gain for all the frequencies was better in the percutaneous group with the most significant gain seen at 4000 Hz. Speech reception threshold values, however, were statistically significant between the groups favoring the percutaneous one.

Complications

In a review of the literature in 2017, Chen and colleagues[16] reported that erythema and pain at the implant site were most common (19%), with resolution of the symptoms in most patients with a decrease in magnet strength. They also reported on 1 case of skin necrosis that was thought to be caused by the use of a strong magnet. Subsequently, the Baha was converted to a percutaneous device. To avoid similar complications, these investigators recommended the use of weaker magnets with restricted daily use in the initial fitting period. Two more cases of skin necrosis in primary Baha Attract patients were later reported.[17]

Other reported complications include seroma or hematoma formation, numbness around the area of the flap, swelling, and detachment of the sound processor from the external magnet.[15]

It is important to note that the use of Baha Attract is to be avoided in patients requiring repeated MRI evaluation of the internal auditory canal area owing to the resultant artifact.

REFERENCES

1. Iseri M, Orhan KS, Tuncer U, et al. Transcutaneous bone-anchored hearing aids versus percutaneous ones: multicenter comparative clinical study. Otol Neurotol 2015;36(5):849–53.
2. Denoyelle F, Coudert C, Thierry B, et al. Hearing rehabilitation with the closed skin bone-anchored implant Sophono Alpha1: results of a prospective study in 15 children with ear atresia. Int J Pediatr Otorhinolaryngol 2015;79(3):382–7.
3. Marsell P, Scorpecci A, Vallarino MV, et al. Sophono in pediatric patients: the experience of an Italian tertiary care center. Otolaryngol Head Neck Surg 2014; 151(2):328–32.
4. O'Neil MB, Runge CL, Friedland DR, et al. Patient Outcomes in Magnet-Based Implantable Auditory Assist Devices. JAMA Otolaryngology Head and Neck Surg 2014;140(6):513–20.
5. Kohan D. Transcutaneous versus Percutaneous Osseointegrated Auditory Implants-Surgical and Audiologic Outcomes, Poster FO30, COSM, Chicago, IL;2016.
6. Nelissen RC, Agterberg MJH, Hol MKS, et al. Three-year experience with the Sophono in children with congenital conductive unilateral hearing loss: tolerability, audiometry, and sound localization compared to a bone-anchored hearing aid. Eur Arch Otorhinolaryngol 2016;273(10):3149–56.
7. Shellock FG. Internal test report, evaluations of magnetic field interactions, hearing and artifacts for the alpha 1 (m) magnetic implant. 2012.
8. Azadarmaki R, Tubbs R, Chen DA, et al. MRI information of commonly used otologic implants: review and update. Otolaryngol Head Neck Surg 2014;150(4):512–9.
9. Hakansson B, Tjellstrom A, Rosenhall U. Hearing thresholds with direct bone conduction versus conventional bone conduction. Scand Audiol 1984;13:3–13.
10. Verstraeten N, Zarowski AJ, Somers T, et al. Comparison of the audiologic results obtained with the bone-anchored hearing aid attached to the headband, the best band, and to the 'snap' abutment. Otol Neurotol 2009;30:70–5.

11. Briggs R, Van Hasselt A, Luntz M, et al. Clinical performance of a new magnetic bone conduction hearing implant system: results from a prospective, multicenter, clinical investigation. Otol Neurotol 2015;36(5):834–41.
12. Hougaard DD, Boldsen SK, Jensen AM, et al. A multicenter study on objective and subjective benefits with a transcutaneous bone-anchored hearing aid device: first Nordic results. Eur Arch Otorhinolaryngol 2017;274:3011–9.
13. Dimitriadis PA, Hind D, Wright K, et al. Single-center experience of over a hundred implantations of a transcutaneous bone conduction device. Otol Neurotol 2017;38(9):1301–7.
14. Cedars E, Chan D, Lao A, et al. Conversion of traditional osseointegrated bone-anchored hearing aids to the Baha® attract in four pediatric patients. Int J Pediatr Otorhinolaryngol 2016;91:37–42.
15. Dimitriadis PA, Farr MR, Allam A, et al. Three year experience with the cochlear BAHA attract implant: a systematic review of the literature. BMC Ear Nose Throat Disord 2016;16:12.
16. Chen SY, Mancuso D, Lalwani AK. Skin necrosis after implantation with the BAHA attract: a case report and review of the literature. Otol Neurotol 2017;38(3):364–7.
17. Nevoux J, Papon JF. RE: skin necrosis after implantation with the Baha Attract: a case report and review of the literature: Chen SY, Mancuso D, and Lalwani AK. Otol Neurotol 2017;38(3): 364-7. Otol Neurotol 2017;38(9):1382–3.

Osseointegrated Auditory Devices: Bonebridge

Mia E. Miller, MD

KEYWORDS

- Bonebridge • Bone conduction device • FMT • Aural atresia

KEY POINTS

- Bonebridge is an active bone conduction device in use in Europe and other countries, and it was recently approved by Food and Drug Administration for use in the United States.
- Bonebridge has indications for use similar to other bone conduction devices, including conductive and mixed hearing loss or single-sided deafness.
- Surgery for Bonebridge placement requires computed tomography scan and planning to create a well for the bone conduction-floating mass transducer; inadequate bone depth or previous surgery may require alterations of the surgical plan.
- Some advantages of Bonebridge include lack of skin complications, no need for osseointegration, and earlier activation.
- Most studies comparing hearing outcomes between Bonebridge and other bone conduction devices demonstrate equivalent outcomes.

INTRODUCTION

Bonebridge (Vibrant MedEl, Innsbruck, Austria) is a device approved for children 5 years and older[1] in most countries, and it very recently received approval from Food and Drug Administration (FDA) for use in the United States for patients 12 years and older. It is a transcutaneous active bone conduction device, which differentiates it from passive bone conduction devices widely used in the United States. Reports from early use in Europe have been favorable in terms of risk of complications, hearing outcomes, and patient satisfaction. Surgery for implantation is straightforward, and indications for use are similar to other bone conduction devices.

DEVICE COMPONENTS

Bonebridge has both internal and external components (**Fig. 1**). The implanted device consists of the bone conduction-floating mass transducer (BC-FMT) and magnet, and the external component is the SAMA audio processor (AP). The AP attaches transcutaneously to the internal component with a magnet and is powered by a hearing aid battery (**Fig. 2**).

No disclosures.
House Clinic, 2100 West 3rd Street, Suite 111, Los Angeles, CA 90057, USA
E-mail address: mmiller@houseclinic.com

Otolaryngol Clin N Am 52 (2019) 265–272
https://doi.org/10.1016/j.otc.2018.11.006
0030-6665/19/© 2018 Elsevier Inc. All rights reserved.

oto.theclinics.com

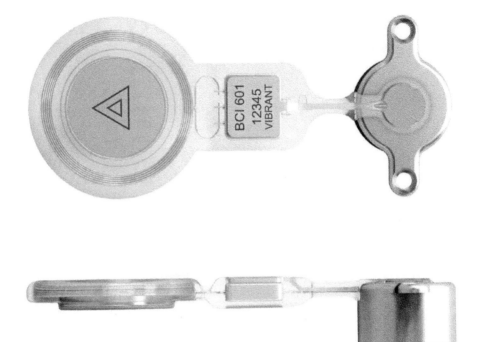

Fig. 1. Bonebridge device viewed from top and side with magnet on left and BC-FMT on right. (*Courtesy of* Med-El Co., Durham, NC; with permission.)

ACTIVE BONE CONDUCTION

The AP detects sound and transmits it to the implant. The BC-FMT then directly vibrates the adjacent bone. This mechanism is different from passive percutaneous

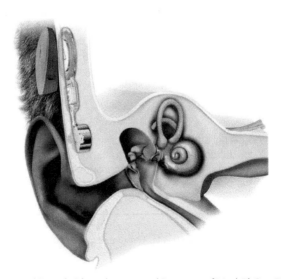

Fig. 2. Ear anatomy and Bonebridge placement. (*Courtesy of* Med-El Co., Durham, NC; with permission.)

bone conduction devices (such as the Baha Connect or Ponto) as well as passive transcutaneous bone conduction devices (such as the Baha Attract and Sophono), because bone conduction is an active process with the FMT.

DEVICE INDICATIONS

The FDA granted Bonebridge de novo clearance for use in patients 12 years and older with conductive hearing loss, mixed hearing loss, or single-sided deafness in July 2018. Bonebridge is indicated internationally in adults and children older than 5 years with a conductive hearing loss (bone pure tone average [PTA] at 0.5, 1, 2, 3, and 4 kHz less than or equal to 45 dB) or with single-sided deafness (SSD) with an air PTA of the hearing ear of 20 dB or better.[2] Computed tomography (CT) should be performed to ascertain that the temporal bone is suitable for FMT placement and patients should be cleared of retrocochlear pathology.

Patients with ear canal atresia are among those with the largest functional gain with Bonebridge implantation because of a relatively large air-bone gap and often normally functioning inner ear.[3] Other indications include ear canal stenosis or a chronic draining ear where a hearing aid cannot be safely fitted, otosclerosis not suitable for stapedectomy, and unrecovered sudden sensorineural hearing loss resulting in SSD.

SURGERY

Bonebridge implant surgery can be done under general or local anesthesia.[4] A 4 cm incision is made 1 cm behind the external auditory canal. A V-shaped flap is then elevated to expose the mastoid bone, and a periosteal pocket is created posterior to this. A sizer is used to mark the anticipated location of the BC-FMT, and a well is drilled 9 mm deep for this part of the device, which is 1 cm in height (**Fig. 3**). The BC-FMT is placed into the well, the coil part of the implant is placed in the periosteal pocket, and the BC-FMT is fixed with cortical osseointegratable screws. The tissues are then closed in a layered fashion.

A CT scan should be used preoperatively to determine the optimal location of the BC-FMT well. The classic location of the BC-FMT well is presigmoid near the sinodural angle.[5] The location of the well should be moved to accommodate anatomy, such as more posteriorly for a patient with a mastoid cavity. According to the published literature, the dura or sigmoid sinus may be exposed and/or compressed during the

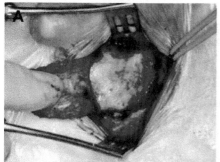
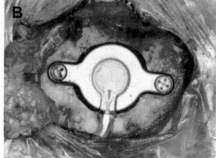

Fig. 3. Intraoperative photos. (*A*) V-shaped periosteal flap. (*B*) Bone conduction implant in place. (*From* Steinmetz C, Mader I, Arndt S, et al. MRI artifacts after bonebridge implantation. Eur Arch Otorhinolaryngol 2014;271:2079–82; with permission.)

procedure. Lifts are now provided by the manufacturer to reduce implantation depth when required, which may reduce the likelihood of dural compression. In patients in whom a presigmoid or retrosigmoid placement is not possible, a "middle fossa" placement has been described, with an incision made above the ear.[6]

In a recent study, CT images of 151 mastoids from children and young adults were examined and found that the mastoid was of adequate size for Bonebridge implantation in most of the adults. However, only 50% of 12 year olds had adequate bone depth for placement of the implant, and 6 year-old patients required lifts for implantation.[7]

Although all surgeons use preoperative CT for BC-FMT planning,[8,9] some have gone further with the creation of a temporal bone well template that demonstrates the well in situ after 3-dimensional (3D) CT analysis.[10,11] Others have described Bonebridge implantation using image guidance,[12] 3D software modeling for surgical planning,[13] and even 3D printed temporal bones for surgical planning.[14,15]

ADVANTAGES AND DISADVANTAGES

With the Bonebridge implant, there is no percutaneous component, so skin infections are not a problem for patients who use them.[16] Lack of the percutaneous component is also desirable aesthetically to both adult and pediatric patients. In addition, it does not require osseointegration, which allows for earlier activation (2–4 weeks) and fewer complications. In bone conduction devices that do require osseointegration, problems with integration and head trauma lead to higher loss rates of fixtures in children than in adults.[17–19]

Where it is approved for usage, Bonebridge is MRI conditional up to 1.5 T with the external component removed, although there is a large artifact due to the internal magnet (**Fig. 4**). The manufacturer indicates that MRI artifact can be up to 15 cm and even affect the magnetic resonance signal of contralateral pathology.[20] Advantages and disadvantages of active compared with passive percutaneous bone conduction devices can be seen in **Table 1**.

OUTCOMES
Safety

A recent systematic review of 12 studies including 117 patients reported complications.[2] Nine of the studies reported no adverse events, whereas others reported minor complications, such as temporary tinnitus and dizziness, headache or wound pain, seroma, and minor wound infection.

In addition to a favorable safety profile, postoperative pain has shown to be comparable between Bonebridge and cochlear implants using a Headache Impact Test.[21]

Hearing Outcomes

A review of 11 studies examining hearing after Bonebridge in patients with conductive or mixed loss demonstrated a functional gain from 24 to 37 dB.[2] Longer-term data after 12 to 18 months of use shows this gain is stable,[22] and other studies demonstrate that patients report subjective benefit that is stable over time.[23]

Hearing benefit has also been demonstrated in patients with SSD, although in smaller studies.[24–26] An increase in speech recognition has been noted especially in complex listening environments in this patient population, such as when noise is presented to the normal hearing ear.[27] Some investigators have also reported a learning curve, with increased speech in noise understanding with longer device use.[28]

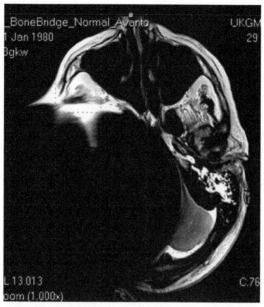

Fig. 4. Example of MRI artifact with Bonebridge in place in the sinodural angle position. (*Courtesy of* C. Güldner, MD, Marburg, Germany; and Med-El Co., Durham, NC, with permission Med-El Co.)

A recent study from Chile demonstrated normal and near-normal thresholds after Bonebridge implantation in a pediatric cohort with atresia and microtia.[29] Others have shown implanted thresholds to be superior to softband Bonebridge thresholds in this patient population.[30] Moreover, as with percutaneous passive bone conduction devices, this active bone conduction device demonstrates more reliable and durable hearing improvement than does aural atresia surgery.[31] It has also provided hearing improvement with other congenital anomalies, such as oval window atresia associated with conductive hearing loss[32] and microtia with stapes ankylosis.[33]

When compared with matched patients with Cochlear Corporation percutaneous Baha devices, patients with Bonebridge demonstrate audiologically equivalent outcomes, with no significant differences in functional gain or word recognition score.[34] Cadaveric studies reveal similar cochlear promontory acceleration between Baha and Bonebridge when measured with laser Doppler vibrometry.[35] Although some studies have reported audiological performance differences when a softband is used,[35] a prospective study comparing implanted Bonebridge with soft-band Baha showed no significant differences.[36] Bonebridge has also been compared with the Sophono device, and they show comparable functional gain (**Box 1**).[37]

Table 1	
Active compared with passive percutaneous devices	
Advantages	**Disadvantages**
Fewer skin complications	Surgical planning for BC-FMT well
No need for osseointegration	May require lifts (higher profile)
Early activation	Artifact on MRI

> **Box 1**
> **Hearing outcomes**
> • Bonebrige is audiologically equivalent to bone conduction devices in use in the United States.

SUMMARY

The Bonebridge is an active bone conduction hearing device that shows favorable outcomes in studies from Europe. Recent FDA approval of Bonebridge provides an alternative to passive bone conduction hearing devices to patients with conductive and mixed hearing loss or single-sided deafness in the United States.

REFERENCES

1. Available at: http://www.medel.com/products-bonebridge/. Accessed July 1, 2018.
2. Sprinzl GM, Wolf-Magele A. The Bonebridge Bone Conduction Hearing Implant: indication criteria, surgery and a systematic review of the literature. Clin Otolaryngol 2016;41(2):131–43.
3. Riss D, Arnoldner C, Baumgartner WD, et al. Indication criteria and outcomes with the Bonebridge transcutaneous bone-conduction implant. Laryngoscope 2014;124(12):2802–6.
4. Baumgartner WD, Hamzavi JS, Böheim K, et al. A new transcutaneous bone conduction hearing implant: short-term safety and efficacy in children. Otol Neurotol 2016;37(6):713–20.
5. Bianchin G, Bonali M, Russo M, et al. Active bone conduction system: outcomes with the Bonebridge transcutaneous device. ORL J Otorhinolaryngol Relat Spec 2015;77(1):17–26.
6. Zernotti ME, Sarasty AB. Active bone conduction prosthesis: bonebridge(TM). Int Arch Otorhinolaryngol 2015;19(4):343–8.
7. Rahne T, Schilde S, Seiwerth I, et al. Mastoid dimensions in children and young adults: consequences for the geometry of transcutaneous bone-conduction implants. Otol Neurotol 2016;37(1):57–61.
8. Law EK, Bhatia KS, Tsang WS, et al. CT pre-operative planning of a new semi-implantable bone conduction hearing device. Eur Radiol 2016;26(6):1686–95.
9. Schilde S, Plontke SK, Rahne T. A three-dimensional geometric-morphometric study to quantify temporal bone growth and its consequences for the success of implanting bone anchored hearing devices. Otol Neurotol 2017;38(5):721–9.
10. Takumi Y, Matsumoto N, Cho B, et al. A clinical experience of 'STAMP' plate-guided Bonebridge implantation. Acta Otolaryngol 2014;134(10):1042–6.
11. Cho B, Matsumoto N, Mori M, et al. Image-guided placement of the Bonebridge™ without surgical navigation equipment. Int J Comput Assist Radiol Surg 2014;9(5):845–55.
12. Kong TH, Park YA, Seo YJ. Image-guided implantation of the Bonebridge™ with a surgical navigation: a feasibility study. Int J Surg Case Rep 2017;30:112–7.
13. Plontke SK, Radetzki F, Seiwerth I, et al. Individual computer-assisted 3D planning for surgical placement of a new bone conduction hearing device. Otol Neurotol 2014;35(7):1251–7.

14. Mukherjee P, Cheng K, Flanagan S, et al. Utility of 3D printed temporal bones in pre-surgical planning for complex BoneBridge cases. Eur Arch Otorhinolaryngol 2017;274(8):3021–8.

15. Pai I, Rojas P, Jiang D, et al. The use of 3D printed external and internal templates for Bonebridge implantation - technical note. Clin Otolaryngol 2017;42(5):1118–20.

16. Schmerber S, Deguine O, Marx M, et al. Safety and effectiveness of the Bone-bridge transcutaneous active direct-drive bone-conduction hearing implant at 1-year device use. Eur Arch Otorhinolaryngol 2017;274(4):1835–51.

17. Lloyd S, Almeyda J, Sirimanna KS, et al. Updated surgical experience with bone-anchored hearing aids in children. J Laryngol Otol 2007;121:826–31.

18. Lee CE, Christensen L, Richter GT, et al. Arkansas BAHA experience: transcalva-rial fixture placement using osseointegration surgical hardware. Otol Neurotol 2011;32:444–7.

19. Zeitoun H, De R, Thompson SD, et al. Osseointegrated implants in the manage-ment of childhood ear abnormalities: with particular emphasis on complications. J Laryngol Otol 2002;116:87–91.

20. Steinmetz C, Mader I, Arndt S, et al. MRI artefacts after bonebridge implantation. Eur Arch Otorhinolaryngol 2014;271:2079–82.

21. Lassaletta L, Calvino M, Zernotti M, et al. Postoperative pain in patients undergo-ing a transcutaneous active bone conduction implant (Bonebridge). Eur Arch Otorhinolaryngol 2016;273(12):4103–10.

22. Sprinzl G, Lenarz T, Ernst A. et al. The Bonebridge new transcutaneous Bone Conduction Hearing Implant: safety and effectiveness data at 12 to 18 months device use. Presented at 2nd Meeting of the European Academy of Otorhinolar-yngology and Head and Neck Surgery, Nice, France, April 27–30, 2013.

23. Ihler F, Volbers L, Blum J, et al. Preliminary functional results and quality of life after implantation of a new bone conduction hearing device in patients with conductive and mixed hearing loss. Otol Neurotol 2014;35:211–5.

24. Honeder C. Evaluation of the MED-EL Bonebridge in single sided deafness using a multisource noise field. Presented at 13th International Conference on Cochlear Implants and Other Implantable Auditory Technologies, Munich, Germany, June 18–21, 2014.

25. Rivas A, Garcia LE, Forero VH, et al. Bonebridge: auditory and quality of life out-comes in conductive, mixed hearing loss and single sided deafness. Presented at 13th International Conference on Cochlear Implants and Other Implantable Auditory Technologies, Munich, Germany, 2014.

26. Salcher R, Zimmermann D, Giere T, et al. Audiological results in SSD with an active transcutaneous bone conduction implant at a retrosigmoidal position. Otol Neurotol 2017;38(5):642–7.

27. Salcher RB, Gerdes T, Giere T, et al. An active bone conduction implant in pa-tients with single-sided deafness. Presented at 13th International Conference on Cochlear Implants and Other Auditory Technologies, Munich, Germany, 2014.

28. Laske RD, Röösli C, Pfiffner F, et al. Functional results and subjective benefit of a transcutaneous bone conduction device in patients with single-sided deafness. Otol Neurotol 2015;36(7):1151–6.

29. Bravo-Torres S, Der-Mussa C, Fuentes-López E. Active transcutaneous bone con-duction implant: audiological results in paediatric patients with bilateral microtia associated with external auditory canal atresia. Int J Audiol 2018;57(1):53–60.

30. Fan X, Wang Y, Wang P, et al. Aesthetic and hearing rehabilitation in patients with bilateral microtia-atresia. Int J Pediatr Otorhinolaryngol 2017;101:150–7.

31. Jovankovičová A, Staník R, Kunzo S, et al. Surgery or implantable hearing devices in children with congenital aural atresia: 25 years of our experience. Int J Pediatr Otorhinolaryngol 2015;79(7):975–9.
32. Kim M. Bonebridge implantation for conductive hearing loss in a patient with oval window atresia. J Int Adv Otol 2015;11(2):163–6.
33. Zanetti D, Di Berardino F. A bone conduction implantable device as a functional treatment option in unilateral microtia with bilateral stapes ankylosis: a report of two cases. Am J Case Rep 2018;19:82–9.
34. Gerdes T, Salcher RB, Schwab B, et al. Comparison of audiological results between a transcutaneous and a percutaneous bone conduction instrument in conductive hearing loss. Otol Neurotol 2016;37(6):685–91.
35. Huber AM, Sim JH, Xie YZ, et al. The Bonebridge: preclinical evaluation of a new transcutaneously-activated bone anchored hearing device. Hear Res 2013;301: 93–9.
36. Ihler F, Blum J, Berger MU, et al. The prediction of speech recognition in noise with a semi-implantable bone conduction hearing system by external bone conduction stimulation with headband: a prospective study. Trends Hear 2016;20 [pii:2331216516669330].
37. Zernotti ME, Di Gregorio MF, Galeazzi P, et al. Comparative outcomes of active and passive hearing devices by transcutaneous bone conduction. Acta Otolaryngol 2016;136(6):556–8.

Ossicle Coupling Active Implantable Auditory Devices: Magnetic Driven System

C.Y. Joseph Chang, MD[a,b,*]

KEYWORDS

- Maxum • MEI • Middle ear implant • Implantable hearing device
- Speech perception gap • Cochlear hearing potential

KEY POINTS

- Hearing aid (HA) use for moderate to severe hearing loss has several limitations, including the occlusion effect and feedback, which limit high-frequency gain.
- Active auditory implants typically have no feedback limitations and can provide improved hearing function compared with HAs.
- The speech perception gap is defined as phonetically balanced maximum word recognition of a word list minus word recognition score with HA.

INTRODUCTION

Despite many years of research, most cases of sensorineural hearing loss (SNHL) still cannot be restored. Although recent molecular techniques show great promise in restoring sensorineural hearing function, the mainstay of alleviating the disabilities associated with SNHL continues to be amplification. There have been great strides made over the past 30 years with developments such as digital signal processing in hearing aids (HAs) and other devices such as cochlear implants (CIs) and osseointegrated implants. Over the past 20 years, active middle ear implant (MEI) devices have been developed to provide an alternative to HAs, which have limitations for patients with moderate to severe hearing loss. (See Sara Lerner's article, "Limitations of Conventional Hearing Aids – Examining Common Complaints and Issues That Can and Cannot Be Remedied," in this issue.) Essentially, the high-frequency hearing gain of HAs in patients may be limited by the issue of acoustic feedback, resulting in some patients failing to achieve the hearing improvement that would be expected

Disclosures: None.
[a] Texas Ear Center, 7900 Fannin, Suite 1800, Houston, TX 77054, USA; [b] Department of Otorhinolaryngology–Head and Neck Surgery, University of Texas McGovern Medical School, Houston, TX, USA
* 7900 Fannin, Suite 1800, Houston, TX 77054.
E-mail address: drchang@texasent.com

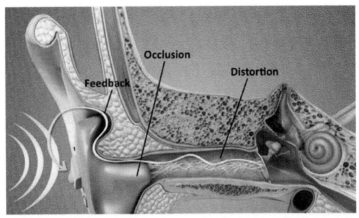

Fig. 1. Cross-section of a HA in the right lateral ear canal and meatus with issues of occlusion effect with resulting distortion and acoustic feedback. (*Courtesy of* Ototronix, LLC, Houston, TX; with permission.)

based on their cochlear hearing potential. These patients typically require closed molds to reduce the feedback issue; however, these occlusive molds can cause the occlusion effect, resulting in sound distortion, autophony, and aural fullness, which many patients find undesirable or even intolerable (**Fig. 1**). To overcome the limitations of HAs, active MEIs have been developed to provide an enhanced hearing experience and function for these patients. There are various devices available on the market today, with different degrees of complexity and cost. This article provides a brief overview of a magnetically driven active implantable auditory device, the Maxum system (Ototronix LLC, St. Paul, MN, USA). It also provides an update on new data that have been published since the last *Otolaryngology Clinics* article on this topic,[1] including an overview of the device, indications, implantation procedure, and outcomes.

DEVICE OVERVIEW

All devices that are used to provide enhanced auditory information to patients are transducers. Essentially, a transducer transforms a signal from 1 form to another. An HA is a sound to sound signal transducer that essentially amplifies without changing the signal medium. A CI is a sound-to-electrical signal transducer to the spiral ganglion. An active MEI is a sound-to-mechanical signal transducer to the ossicular chain. It turns an acoustic signal traveling through air into a mechanical signal that travels through ossicular motions.[2]

The Maxum device is a semi-implantable system that consists of a magnet that is applied to the incudostapedial (IS) joint with a nitinol wire loop and an external in-the-canal (ITC) processor (**Fig. 2**). The ITC processor transforms the incoming sound signal into an electromagnetic signal that drives the magnet using magnetic induction, thereby imparting the corresponding mechanical signal onto the ossicular chain. Because the output signal of the MEI is not a sound signal, there is very little chance of acoustic feedback that could limit high-frequency gain. The lack of significant feedback issue allows the Maxum external processor to have a large-bore vent that prevents the occlusion effect so that patients do not experience the disturbing sound distortion, autophony, and aural fullness (**Fig. 3**). It can, therefore, deliver a much larger

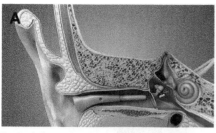
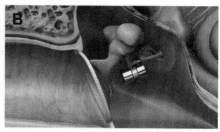

Fig. 2. (*A*) Cross-section of the Maxum system in the right ear canal consisting of an ITC processor and a separate magnetic implant attached to the IS joint. (*B*) Cross-section of the Maxum magnet attached to the IS joint. (*Courtesy of* Ototronix, LLC, Houston, TX; with permission.)

high-frequency gain in real world use compared with HAs without many of the side effects associated with an HA closed mold.

SELECTION CRITERIA

The Maxum is approved for use by the US Food and Drug Administration and is indicated for patients with moderate to severe SNHL who are not benefiting adequately with properly fitted HAs. Patients should be 18 years or older, have no tympanic membrane (TM) perforation, middle ear or mastoid disease, conductive component of hearing loss, or retrocochlear disease on the side of implantation. The Maxum MEI is not safe for MRI. The speech discrimination score should be 60% or higher.

The audiometric profile for Maxum candidacy (**Fig. 4**A) shows that it is indicated for patients with moderate to severe hearing loss in the HA range and also in the CI range. Indeed, close inspection of the Maxum audiometric profile shows that it significantly overlaps with criteria for standard and hybrid CIs (**Fig. 4**B). Therefore, there may be some difficulty determining whether a particular candidate for a CI may also benefit from MEI and, therefore, be a potential candidate for either device. In addition, there may be some difficulty determining whether a patient with hearing loss in the HA range may do better with the Maxum.

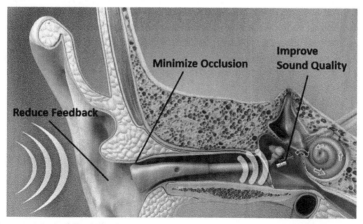

Fig. 3. Cross-section of the Maxum system in the right lateral ear canal with lack of occlusion effect (due to a large-bore vent within the mold) and lack of feedback (related to the lack of acoustic signal output). (*Courtesy of* Ototronix, LLC, Houston, TX; with permission.)

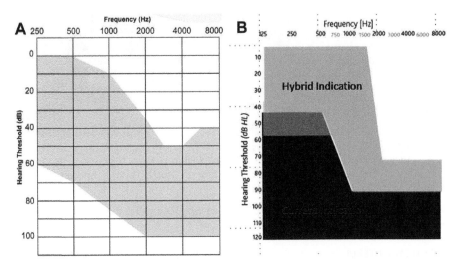

Fig. 4. (*A*) Audiogram profile for the Maxum. (*B*) Audiogram profile for the standard CI (current indication) and hybrid CI. Note that there is a large overlap between the Maxum and CI profiles, indicating that there will be patients who are candidates for both the Maxum and CI. dB HL, decibel hearing loss. (*Courtesy of* [A] Ototronix, LLC, Houston, TX; with permission.)

The MEI preserves the patient's native hearing function as opposed to CI with which most patients lose all of their native hearing function or incur a significant decrease in native hearing function. In addition, the overall cost of the Maxum is much lower than that of the CI, although insurance coverage for MEI is less certain that for CI. There is significant interest in identifying patients considered for a CI who would also do well with an MEI, which may then be offered as a viable, nondestructive hearing option. Recent work has shown a method of identifying CI candidate patients who may also obtain very good hearing results with the Maxum. In addition, this work has shown a method of identifying patients who may obtain better word recognition scores (WRSs) with the Maxum than with their best fitted HA and to estimate the degree of hearing improvement with the Maxum compared with the HA (see later discussion).

Although many patients with moderate to severe SNHL attain their cochlear hearing potential using well fitted HAs, a significant number of patients fail to achieve this level of hearing function (**Fig. 5**).[3] Each patient's cochlear hearing potential may be estimated by the phonetically balanced maximum (PB Max) word recognition of a word list, which estimates the maximum WRS feasible based on the degree of cochlear damage because the testing is done in ideal noise-free circumstances using earphones. Word discrimination testing using HAs can then be performed to see if the WRS using the HA is close to the PB Max. If the WRS using HAs is significantly less than the PB Max, there is a speech perception gap (SPG), defined as the PB Max minus WRS using HAs. The Maxum MEI can provide patients a WRS much closer to the PB Max, so the SPG can predict the expected magnitude of improved speech understanding with the Maxum MEI over HAs for a particular patient.[4]

PRESURGICAL EVALUATION

The Maxum MEI ITC processor is a deep insertion device that requires the creation of a custom-fitted mold. Similar to the OtoLens, the impression is taken deep down to and including the lateral surface marks of the TM. There are some patients whose

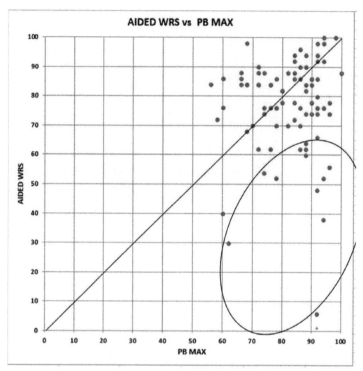

Fig. 5. Scatter plot of HA users who were subjects of the Maxum US Food and Drug Administration study showing that the WRS using HAs are close to the PB Max line (cochlear hearing potential) but that a subset of subjects scored significantly below their PB Max score, indicating HAs were underperforming their cochlear hearing potential (*circled area*). PB Max, phonetically balanced maximum (word recognition of word list). (*Courtesy of* Ototronix, LLC, Houston, TX; with permission.)

external auditory canals (EACs) may look acceptable but are actually too tortuous for proper fitting of the processor. These patients are identified when the deep ear canal impression is inspected by the manufacturer. The patient will also need a general evaluation of their manual dexterity to ensure that they are able to manipulate the ITC processor as is standard for ITC HA evaluations.

SURGICAL TECHNIQUE

The surgery for implantation of the MEI magnet uses an approach similar to stapedectomy. A transcanal approach, including raising of the tympanomeatal flap, is performed. An adequate amount of scutum removal to visualize the horizontal course of the facial nerve and the pyramidal process is needed. The MEI magnet is then positioned just inferior to the IS joint and the nitinol wire loop is placed around the IS joint and closed around the joint using either a laser or heating element (**Figs. 6–8**). Occasionally, an additional manual crimp of the wire loop is needed. The loop will not tighten onto the ossicles as a stapes implant wire loop does, so proper fixation to the ossicular chain requires application of an otologic cement (**Fig. 9**).

  The glass ionomer cement (Procem) has a working time of 1 to 2 minutes after it is mixed. This duration may be extended somewhat by keeping it cool on an ice pack

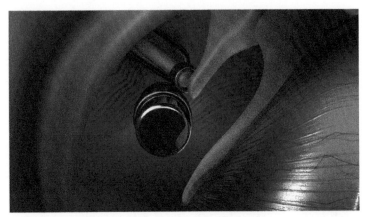

Fig. 6. The Maxum magnet implant attached to the IS joint for the right ear in surgical position. The magnet is placed close to its final position before application of the cement. (*Courtesy of* Ototronix, LLC, Houston, TX; with permission.)

covered with sterile plastic on the surgical field just before application. During the working time, the cement is applied around the wire loop and IS joint. The MEI typically moves out of proper position during this portion of the procedure and must be repositioned during the cement working period. It is helpful to apply a piece of Gelfoam onto the promontory inferior to the MEI magnet to stabilize it in position before application of the cement. After the end of the cement working time, the cure time for adequate fixation is an additional 6 minutes, and it reaches most of its strength and stability at 24 hours after surgery.

During the cement application, care must be taken to avoid applying the cement anywhere else in the middle ear, especially along the facial nerve because the cement is neurotoxic. In addition, inadvertent cement application to other areas of the ossicular chain could result in ossicular fixation if the cement also fixates to surrounding structures. The MEI positioning is also highly critical as the magnet must be in close alignment with the axis of the EAC. This is accomplished by positioning the MEI so

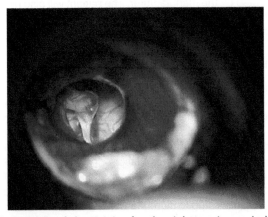

Fig. 7. Surgical photograph of the IS joint for the right ear in surgical position showing proper surgical exposure.

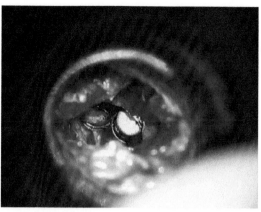

Fig. 8. Surgical photograph of the Maxum magnetic implant after crimping to the IS joint for the right ear in surgical position. (*Courtesy of* Ototronix, LLC, Houston, TX.)

that the lateral face of the implant directly faces the longitudinal axis of the EAC (see **Fig. 9**). Improper positioning of the MEI magnet during implantation will result in decreased functional gain due to misalignment between the MEI magnet and the magnetic field created by the processor. Also, the MEI magnet must not contact the TM, which could lead to TM perforation and MEI exposure, and it also must not contact the promontory.

After the MEI has been adequately installed, the tympanomeatal flap is replaced back in position. Photographs of the MEI before and after TM replacement are taken with the microscope in the same position to provide to the company (**Fig. 10**). This information will be used when manufacturing the external processor so that the processor tip, which produces the magnetic signal, is in proper alignment to the MEI magnetic axis. This manufacturing process cannot fully compensate for a grossly misaligned MEI magnet. Postoperative care is similar to that after any transcanal ear

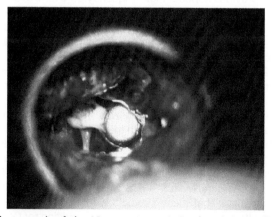

Fig. 9. Surgical photograph of the Maxum magnetic implant joint in final position after application of the surgical cement to the wire loop and IS for the right ear in surgical position. Note that the anterior face of the magnet faces directly to the surgeon's view, indicating proper magnet orientation. (*Courtesy of* Ototronix, LLC, Houston, TX.)

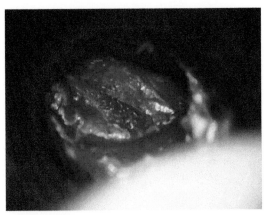

Fig. 10. Surgical photograph of the TM taken in the same position as in **Fig. 9** after the tympanomeatal flap is replaced.

surgery. The initial processor fitting and programming can be performed about a month after surgery.

OUTCOMES

The possible postsurgical complications include MEI exposure, MEI loosening due to failure of the cement or ossicular erosion, and other standard risks associated with transcanal ear surgery. The incidence of these complications is thought to be very low; however, the actual complication rates have not been published to date. There have also been no reports of severe SNHL related to the surgery or the device to date. The effect of mass loading of the ossicular chain due to the MEI magnet may cause a 4 dB conductive hearing loss on average in some patients. The long-term stability of MEI magnet attachment or dislocation with ossicle erosion after prolonged use has not been determined.

The Maxum MEI provides superior high-frequency pure tone average (HFPTA) (2, 3, and 4 kHz) gain compared with HAs in patients who are not achieving their cochlear hearing potential with HA use. In a study by Chang and colleagues,[4] 11 subjects with moderate to severe hearing loss who were dissatisfied with HAs were evaluated. The average Maxum HFPTA gain was 39.8 dB (range 21.7–50.0 dB, median 43.3 dB) compared with 22.7 dB (range 6.7–41.7 dB, median 23.3 dB) with HAs. The average WRS was 65% (range 28%–94%, median 64%) with the MEI compared with 23% (range 0%–84%, median 64%) with HAs. Similarly, in a study by Hunter and colleagues,[5] the average Maxum HFPTA gain was 47.2 dB compared with 22.5 dB with HAs. The average WRS was 81.5% with the MEI compared with 39.5% with HAs.

A subset of subjects who were probable CI candidates in the former Maxum study,[4] with WRSs less than 30% using HAs, who also had PB Max scores of 60% or higher, were analyzed separately. In this group of 7 subjects, the average WRS with HAs was 14.9%, whereas the average Maxum WRS was 67.4% (range 58%–82%, median 64%). These results show that these subjects would no longer be CI candidates if Maxum hearing results were used as the best aided condition for CI evaluation. These WRS results[6] also compare favorably to a CI study by Gifford and colleagues[6] that showed similar average WRS results with the CI. In this study, the CI subjects actually had better average HA WRS than those of the subjects in the Maxum study, implying

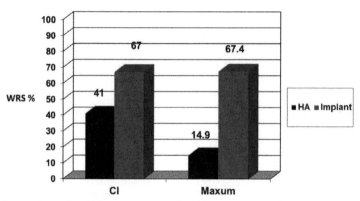

Fig. 11. Comparison of WRS between HA and CI (6) versus HA and Maxum. (4) The Maxum WRS are comparable to the CI WRS, even though the HA scores in the Maxum patients were lower than the HA scores of CI patients, indicating Maxum patients had worse native hearing than the CI patients. CNC, consonant-nucleus-consonant word test. (*Courtesy of* Ototronix, LLC, Houston, TX.)

that the MEI subjects had worse underlying hearing function compared with the CI subjects. Despite this potential disadvantage, the average Maxum WRS was similar to the average CI WRS (**Fig. 11**).

Patient survey data were also presented in the Chang and colleagues[4] study. Abbreviated Profile of Hearing Aid Benefit scores showed improvement with the Maxum over HAs in the ease of communication and background noise subscales, whereas reverberation and aversiveness remained unchanged. However, these differences were not statistically significant. A patient preference survey showed a significant patient preference for the Maxum over HAs in this population (**Table 1**). The average score for the 10 items evaluating performance during different listening conditions was 4.3 (of 5) (range 2.6–5.0, median 4.4) in favor of the MEI over HAs.

Table 1
Maxum system hearing device preference system results (*N* = 10)

	Average	Minimum	Maximum	Median
Sound Quality	4.5	2	5	5
Naturalness of Own Voice	4.3	3	5	4
Feedback	3.9	2	5	4
Speech in Noise	3.9	1	5	4
Speech in Car	4.5	4	5	4.5
Speech with Multiple Talkers	3.9	1	5	4
Speech in Quiet	4.7	4	5	5
Music	4.1	1	5	4
Wind Noise	4.1	2	5	4
Device Preference	4.7	4	5	5

*Scale: 5, Maxum much better; 4, Maxum better; 3, neutral; 2, HA better; 1, HA much better.

From Chang CYJ, Spearman M, Spearman B, et al. Comparison of an electromagnetic middle ear implant and hearing aid word recognition performance to word recognition performance obtained under earphones. Otol Neurotol 2017;38(9):1308–14; with permission.

As previously mentioned, the Maxum WRS results more closely match the patient's PB Max score, which is the best WRS using earphones under ideal conditions. Chang and colleagues[4] showed that in a group of subjects with moderate to severe SNHL who are dissatisfied with HA use, the correlation between the Maxum WRS and PB Max was quite high and statistically significant ($r = 0.85$, $P = .001$), whereas the correlation between the HA WRS and PB Max was moderate and not statistically significant ($R = 0.49$, $P = .126$) (**Fig. 12**). The high correlation between PB Max and Maxum WRS has also been shown in another series of subjects by Dyer and colleagues.[7]

The poor correlation between PB Max and WRSs using HAs in this patient group results in an SPG, defined as PB Max minus WRS using HAs. The average SPG using HAs in the Chang and colleagues[4] study was 48.2% (range 6%–76%, median 54%). In comparison, the average SPG using Maxum was 6.6% (range 8%–23%, median 6%), a 41.6% improvement over HAs. The SPG, therefore, quantifies the degree to which HAs are underperforming the patient's cochlear hearing potential. The SPG can also estimate the magnitude of WRS improvement with the MEI compared with HAs and would be of significant clinical benefit in identifying proper candidates for the Maxum MEI and in counseling patients regarding their estimated hearing improvement with the Maxum compared with the HA.

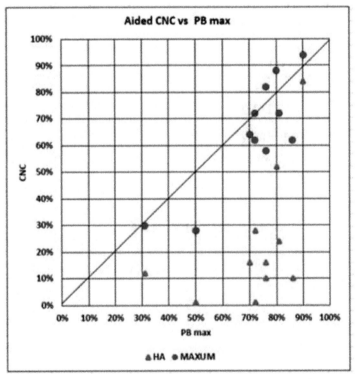

Fig. 12. CNC WRS versus PB max. The PB Max is the diagonal line. Note that most of the HA WRS are clustered around the PB Max line but some, noted by the circle, fall significantly below the PB Max line, indicating that these patients are performing significantly below their cochlear hearing potential with HA use. (*From* Chang CYJ, Spearman M, Spearman B, et al. Comparison of an electromagnetic middle ear implant and hearing aid word recognition performance to word recognition performance obtained under earphones. Otol Neurotol 2017;38(9):1308–14; with permission.)

SUMMARY

The Maxum MEI is among the most straightforward active implantable auditory devices available today. It consists of a magnetic implant attached to the IS joint and an external ITC processor. It alleviates the occlusion effect with a large-bore vent in the processor mold. The implantation process consists of a transcanal approach similar to stapedectomy.

The Maxum MEI can provide a significantly larger amount of HFPTA gain compared with HAs in certain patients due to the lack of acoustic feedback with the MEI. Patients who show a significant SPG, which can be determined by their PB Max and WRS using HAs, are expected to perform significantly better with the Maxum compared with HAs. Patients with PB Max scores of 60% or higher are likely good candidates for this MEI. The degree of WRS improvement with Maxum over HAs may be estimated by the SPG as well. The final Maxum WRS may be estimated to be close to the PB Max. Patients with PB Max scores significantly lower than 60% may be better candidates for the CI because the MEI performance is limited by the patient's underlying cochlear hearing potential.

The calculation of the SPG for patients with HAs who are dissatisfied with their HA performance will likely be a useful tool for evaluating not only the efficacy of HAs and the Maxum MEI but also for other amplification devices. Additional studies are needed to evaluate the benefit of SPG as a tool for other hearing devices. Future larger and longer term studies of the performance of the Maxum MEI will be highly valuable because the currently available data were obtained from a relatively small cohort of subjects.

REFERENCES

1. Pelosi S, Carlson ML, Glasscock ME 3rd. Implantable hearing devices: the Ototronix MAXUM system. Otolaryngol Clin North Am 2014;47(6):953–65.
2. Chang CYJ. Middle ear hearing devices. In: De Souza C, editor. Otorhinolaryngology head and neck surgery. 2nd edition. London: JP Medical Ltd; 2017. p. 2156–64.
3. McRacken T, Ahlstrom J, Clinkscales W, et al. Clinical implications of word recognition differences in earphone and aided conditions. Otol Neurotol 2016;37: 1475–81.
4. Chang CYJ, Spearman M, Spearman B, et al. Comparison of an electromagnetic middle ear implant and hearing aid word recognition performance to word recognition performance obtained under earphones. Otol Neurotol 2017;38(9):1308–14.
5. Hunter JB, Carlson ML, Glasscock ME 3rd. The Ototronix MAXUM middle ear implant for severe high-frequency sensorineural hearing loss: preliminary results. Laryngoscope 2016;126(9):2124–7.
6. Gifford RH, Dorman MF, Shallop JK, et al. Evidence for the expansion of adult cochlear implant candidacy. Ear Hear 2010;31(2):186–94.
7. Dyer RK, Spearman M, Spearman B, et al. Evaluating speech perception of the MAXUM middle ear implant versus speech perception under inserts. Laryngoscope 2018;128(2):456–60.

The Vibrant Soundbridge
A Global Overview

Jennifer Maw, MD, FRCS(C)[a,b,*]

KEYWORDS

- Vibrant Soundbridge • Implantable hearing device
- Surgical treatment of hearing loss

KEY POINTS

- The Vibrant Soundbridge is a semi-implantable, active middle ear implant.
- This device is an effective and safe alternative for the treatment of sensorineural hearing loss.
- It is used internationally for the treatment of conductive and mixed hearing losses of all types.
- It is currently under investigation for conductive and mixed loss in the United States.

INTRODUCTION

The Vibrant Soundbridge (VSB) hearing device (Med-El, Innsbruck, Austria) is an active middle ear implant (AMEI) that was first introduced in the United States and Europe in 1996. It was found to be safe and effective for patients with moderate to severe sensorineural hearing loss (SNHL).[1–4] In the United States, third-party reimbursement for device and surgical costs varies, which has presented challenges to widespread use. There has been extensive expansion of its use globally.

IMPLANT DESCRIPTION

This semi-implantable device (**Fig. 1**) consists of an externally worn audio processor (AP) and the implanted vibrating ossicular replacement prosthesis (VORP) that consists of the floating mass transducer (FMT) and a receiver stimulator (RS) that are connected via a conductor link. The FMT (**Fig. 2**) weighs 25 mg and consists of an electromagnetic coil that surrounds a small magnet.

Similar to a cochlear implant, the AP receives the acoustic signal and modulates and converts it to an electric signal that is passed via radiofrequency to the RS. Current is

Disclosure Statement: None.
[a] Department of Otolaryngology Head and Neck Surgery, Stanford University, Stanford, California; [b] Ear Associates and Rehabilitation Services, Inc., San Jose, California
* Ear Associates and Rehabilitation Services, Inc., 3071 Payne Ave, San Jose, CA 94028.
E-mail address: jlm@earassociates.com

Otolaryngol Clin N Am 52 (2019) 285–295
https://doi.org/10.1016/j.otc.2018.11.007
0030-6665/19/© 2018 Elsevier Inc. All rights reserved.

oto.theclinics.com

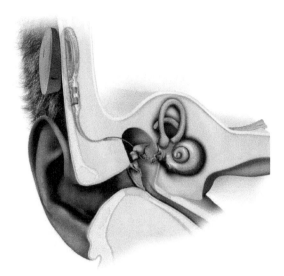

Fig. 1. The implanted Med-El Vibrant Soundbridge, VORP502 with the externally worn AP. (*Courtesy of* Med-El Co, Durham, NC; with permission.)

delivered to the electromagnetic coil, and the inertial mass of the magnet results in a reactive force on the casing, causing its vibratory movement. The FMT can be coupled anywhere along the nascent ossicular chain, attached to or inserted as a middle ear prosthesis, placed on the oval window (OW), round window (RW), or on a fenestrated area of the promontory. In the United States, the current Food and Drug Administration

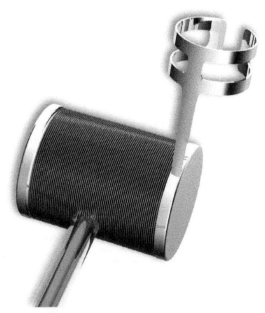

Fig. 2. The FMT. (*Courtesy of* Med-El Co, Durham, NC; with permission.)

(FDA)-approved indication couples the FMT to the long process of the incus to treat SNHL, although a clinical trial is in process to support RW placement for conductive hearing loss (CHL) and mixed hearing loss (MHL) as other approved indications. A variety of other coupling options described in later discussion are successfully in use elsewhere in the world.

VIBRANT SOUNDBRIDGE ADVANTAGES IN SENSORINEURAL HEARING LOSS

- Natural sound quality
- Open ear canal
- No feedback, distortion, occlusion
- Improved speech discrimination in noise
- Improved aesthetics over visible hearing aids

PATIENT CRITERIA FOR SENSORINEURAL HEARING LOSS

- Stable moderate to severe SNHL (**Fig. 3**)
- No middle ear disease, normal immittance
- Speech discrimination >50%
- Healthy scalp at AP site

INDICATIONS FOR SENSORINEURAL HEARING LOSS

- Ear canal problems
- Side effects from hearing aid use
- Dissatisfaction with hearing aid sound quality/cosmesis

SURGERY FOR SENSORINEURAL HEARING LOSS

The RS is implanted as in cochlear implant surgery (**Fig. 4**). In the United States (VORP 502; **Fig. 5**A), the opening of the facial recess must be generous to allow for crimping

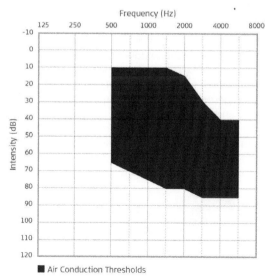

Fig. 3. Audiometric criteria for VSB treatment of SNHL. (*Courtesy of* Med-El Co, Durham, NC.)

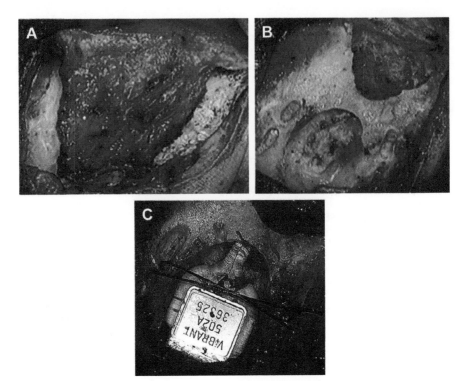

Fig. 4. (*A*) The periosteum is opened as an anteriorly based Palva flap. (*B*) A recessed bed and suture retention holes are drilled. A bony bridge at the edge of the mastoid cavity protects the conductor link. (*C*) The RS is secured with nonabsorbable suture.

of the clip of the FMT to the incus long process (**Fig. 6**). In 2014, the VORP 503 (**Fig. 5**B) was released in international markets. It features a thinner implant design, fixation wings for self-drilling screws, and a shorter and more robust conductor link. The FMT is without a titanium clip and is placed with one of several titanium couplers (**Fig. 7**) to a vibratory structure of the middle ear. In SNHL, it can be crimped on the incus long process (Incus-SMPX-Coupler) or attached without crimping to the long process (Incus-LP-Coupler) or to the incus short process (Incus-SP-Coupler).

Large series[5–7] have demonstrated stable preoperative and postoperative bone conduction thresholds and speech discrimination, good functional gain, and long-term safety.[8–10] Taste loss has been reported from 2% to 6%.[1,9] Aural fullness is a common complication[3] but often resolves. Erosion of the long process has been reported in devices crimped to the incus,[11] but device failure was significantly lower

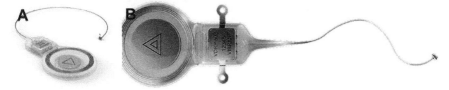

Fig. 5. (*A*) VORP 502 (available in United States). (*B*) VORP 503 (available internationally). (*Courtesy of* Med-El Co, Durham, NC; with permission.)

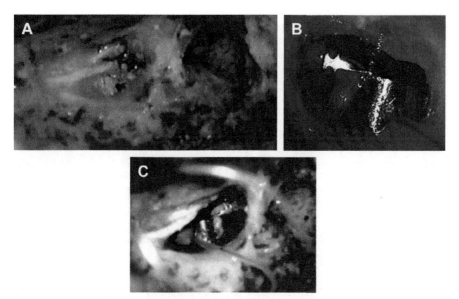

Fig. 6. Placement of the FMT. (*A*) Opening the facial recess. (*B*) Right ear, crimped to incus LP and snug against stapes. (*C*) Left ear. The conductor link should not touch the edges of the facial recess.

when compared with other AMEIs.[11] Device failure has been reported at 7% to 9%[11,12] and was higher in older series using the VORP 501. Longitudinal studies show stable long-term bone conduction thresholds and that implantation of the VSB is atraumatic to residual hearing.[8,9,12–14] **Fig. 8** demonstrates the author's results

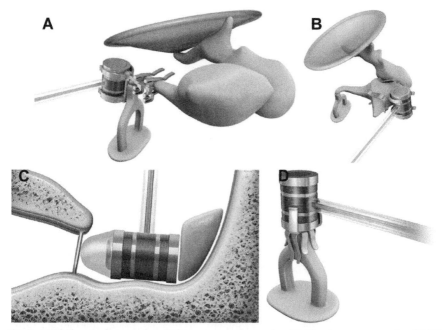

Fig. 7. Med-El ossicular couplers. (*A*) Long process coupler. (*B*) Short process coupler. (*C*) RW coupler. (*D*) Clip coupler. (*Courtesy of* Med-El Co, Durham, NC; with permission.)

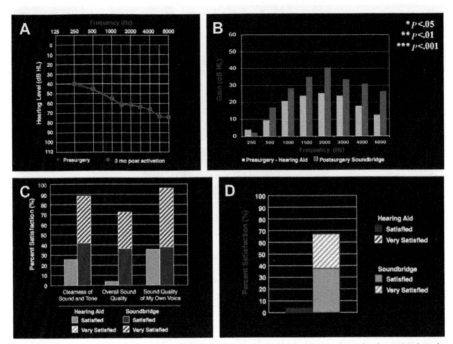

Fig. 8. Preoperative and postoperative results in 22 ears implanted with the VSB by the author. (A) Unaided hearing showing no significant change in residual hearing. (B) The functional gain of VSB compared with hearing aid use. (C) Abbreviated profile of hearing aid benefit results for sound clearness, quality, own voice, and (D) overall satisfaction of hearing aid compared with VSB. HL, hearing loss.

in 22 ears implanted for SNHL showing stable residual hearing, excellent functional gain, and high patient satisfaction.

PATIENT CRITERIA FOR CONDUCTIVE HEARING LOSS AND MIXED HEARING LOSS

- Stable bone conduction thresholds (**Fig. 9**)
- Speech discrimination greater than 50%
- Medically unable to wear acoustic hearing aid
- Inadequate benefit/functional gain from hearing aid

SURGERY FOR CONDUCTIVE HEARING LOSS AND MIXED HEARING LOSS

Hearing results in chronic ear surgery often remain unsatisfactory, and amplification with acoustic hearing aids can be insufficient or cause infection. Percutaneous osseointegrated bone-anchored hearing aids, although surgically simple, are frequently rejected by patients, require significant care, and are associated with long-term complications. Expansion of the VSB indications was therefore desirable. Vibrometer studies had demonstrated similar cochlear fluid movement with vibration of the OW and RW, with a phase difference of about 180°.[15,16]

In 2006, Colletti and colleagues[17] pioneered VSB surgery for CHL and MHL by coupling the FMT to the RW, "RW Vibroplasty," to directly deliver vibrational energy to the scala tympani. Their series demonstrated that the VSB could be implanted in

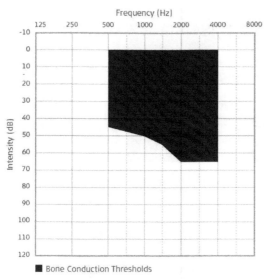

Fig. 9. Audiometric criteria for CHL and MHL.

previously diseased ears without ossicles and poor Eustachian tube function. Placement of the FMT on the RW requires less gain, and patients experience less distortion than with acoustic hearing aids at high volumes. A comparison study of 19 patients with conductive and mixed loss undergoing RW Vibroplasty were compared with patients who had conventional total ossicular replacement prosthesis reconstruction showing significantly improved hearing in the Vibroplasty group.[18]

Safety of the VSB was later shown in the presence of a mastoid cavity in a series of subtotal petrosectomy and obliteration with fat.[19] Other investigators have shown RW Vibroplasty to be safe and effective in chronic ear disease[13,19,20] with stable preoperative to postoperative bone conduction scores. Complications include exposure of the conductor link in the ear canal if not adequately covered with tissue (fascia, cartilage, or allograft). Drilling a trough for the conductor link[21] and covering it with bone pate were also advised.[22] The author has over-closed the ear canal in 2 patients with large mastoid cavities to preclude extrusion issues.

Coupling of the FMT to the RW requires careful removal of the bony overhang and air cells in the hypotympanum to ensure optimal positioning and stability against the RW (**Fig. 10**A). In the US clinical trial, the FMT is coupled to the RW with fascia. Optimal coupling takes experience because of the variability of the RW, and cartilage grafts are sometimes required at the inferior surface of the FMT to support it and prevent decoupling from the RW[23] (**Fig. 10**B, C). Long-term results of this technique are pending. Revision surgery rates in international series ranged from 9.5%[13] to 70% (5/7)[24] in early series. The RW Coupler (Med-El; see **Fig. 7**) device has been devised for improved and more consistent coupling of the FMT to the RW, but long-term studies are pending.

CHL and MHL due to otosclerosis[25] and congenital aural ear atresia[26–29] have also been successfully treated with RW-Vibroplasty. Colletti and colleagues[30] also placed the FMT on a fenestrated area of the promontory patients with OW aplasia, but returned to RW placement due to more stable bone conduction. Improved speech perception and quality of life have been shown with RW Vibroplasty for CHL and MHL when compared with acoustic amplification.[25,31–33] The VSB was also found to

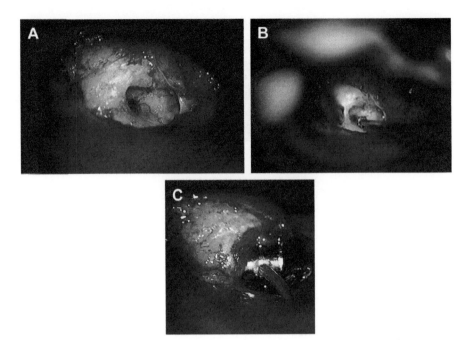

Fig. 10. Surgery for MHL in a mastoid cavity. (*A*) RW exposed. (*B*) Removal of bony over-hang. (*C*) FMT coupled to RW using fascia.

be safe and effective in a series of 19 children with conductive and mixed losses of varied causes,[34] and in atresia, hearing benefit was not observed to be dependent on the Jahrsdoerfer Score.

The FMT was then coupled to any residual vibrating structure in chronic ear surgery, and procedure names were coined, including the stapes head in "Clip Vibroplasty,"[35] the OW niche,[36] the footplate in "Footplate Vibroplasty,"[37] the incus during stapes surgery in "Power Stapes,"[38,39] to a partial or total ossicular replacement prosthesis in "PORP/TORP Vibroplasty,"[37,40,41] or through a perforated fixed footplate in "Direct Oval Window Vibroplasty."[42] The variable demands of the altered anatomy in chronic ear surgery led to the advent of the modified VSB (VORP 503) and coupling devices to facilitate multiple vibroplasty techniques (see **Fig. 7**). The long-term results (4.5–5.6 years) of TORP Vibroplasty using an OW coupler and cartilage shoe on the footplate and cartilage on top of the FMT showed stable functional gain and patient satisfaction over the average 5-year follow-up period.[43] This technique allows passive function as a routine TORP when the sound processor is not worn.

SUMMARY

The VSB is a versatile device for the treatment of SNHL, CHL, and MHL in patients with normal and abnormal anatomy. In the United States, it is FDA approved for SNHL in patients 18 years and older and has been found to be a safe and effective alternative to traditional hearing aids. Longitudinal studies show safety and device stability. There is a great international body of research with expansion of indications. It is C-marked for SNHL, CHL, and mixed hearing loss down to age 3 in Europe. Coupling the VORP to a normal ossicular chain or an ossicular remnant shows good long-term hearing results. RW results show safety of residual hearing. Long-term studies on optimal RW coupling techniques are pending.

REFERENCES

1. Fisch U, Cremers CW, Lenarz T, et al. Clinical experience with the Vibrant Sound-bridge implant device. Otol Neurotol 2001;22(6):962–72.
2. Snik AF, Mylanus EA, Cremers CW, et al. Multicenter audiometric results with the Vibrant Soundbridge, a semi-implantable hearing device for sensorineural hearing impairment. Otolaryngol Clin North Am 2001;34(2):373–88.
3. Luetje C, Brackman D, Balkany T, et al. clinical trial results with the Vibrant Sound-bridge implantable middle ear hearing device: a prospective controlled multicenter study. Otolaryngol Head Neck Surg 2002;126(2):97–107.
4. Arnold A, Stieger C, Candreia C, et al. Factors improving the vibration transfer of the floating mass transducer at the round window. Otol Neurotol 2010;31(1): 122–8.
5. Labassi S, Beliaeff M. Retrospective of 1000 patients implanted with a vibrant Soundbridge middle-ear implant. Cochlear Implants Int 2005;6(Suppl 1):74–7.
6. Sterkers O, Boucarra D, Labassi S, et al. A middle ear implant, the Symphonix Vibrant Soundbridge: retrospective study of the first 125 patients implanted in France. Otol Neurotol 2003;24(3):427–36.
7. Fraysse B, Lavieille JP, Schmerber S, et al. A multicenter study of the Vibrant Soundbridge middle ear implant: early clinical results and experience. Otol Neurotol 2001;22(6):952–61.
8. Vincent C, Fraysse B, Lavieille J, et al. A longitudinal study on postoperative hearing thresholds with the Vibrant Soundbridge device. Eur Arch Otorhinolaryngol 2004;261(9):493–6.
9. Schmuziger N, Schimmann F, Wengen D, et al. Long-term assessment after implantation of the Vibrant Soundbridge device. Otol Neurotol 2006;27(2):183–8.
10. Luetje CM, Brown SA, Cullen RD. Vibrant Soundbridge implantable hearing device: critical review and single-surgeon short- and long-term results. Ear Nose throat J 2010;89(9):E9–14.
11. Zwartenkot JW, Snik AF, Cremers CW, et al. Active middle ear implantation: long-term medical and technical and complications. Otol Neurotol 2016;37(5):513–9.
12. Mosnier I, Sterkers O, Bouccara D, et al. Benefit of the Vibrant Soundbridge device in patients implanted for 5 to 8 years. Ear Hear 2008;29(2):281–4.
13. Skarzynski H, Olszewski L, Skarzynski PH, et al. Direct round window stimulation with the Med-El Vibrant Soundbridge: 5 years of experience using a technique without interposed fascia. Eur Arch Otorhinolaryngol 2014;271(3):477–82.
14. Lenarz T, Weber B, Issing P, et al. Vibrant Sound Bridge System. A new kind hearing prosthesis for patients with sensorineural hearing loss 2 Audiological results. Laryngorhinootologie 2001;80(7):370–80.
15. Ball GR, Huber A, Goode RL. Scanning laser Doppler vibrometry of the middle ear ossicles. Ear Nose Throat J 1997;76(4):213–8, 220, 222.
16. Stenfelt S, Hato N, Goode RL. Round window membrane motion with air conduction and bone conduction stimulation. Hear Res 2004;198(1–2):10–24.
17. Colletti V, Soli S, Carner M, et al. Treatment of mixed hearing losses via implantation of a vibratory transducer on the round window. Int J Audiol 2006;45(10): 600–8.

18. Colletti V, Carner M, Colletti L. TORP vs round window implant for hearing resto-ration of patients with extensive ossicular chain defect. Acta Otolaryngol 2009; 129(4):449–52.

19. Linder T, Schlegel C, DeMin N, et al. van Active middle ear implants in patients undergoing subtotal petrosectomy: new application for the Vibrant Soundbridge device and its implication for lateral cranium base surgery. Otol Neurotol 2009; 30(1):41–7.

20. Baumgartner W, Hagen R, Lenarz T, et al. The vibrant soundbridge for conductive and mixed hearing losses: European multicenter study results. Adv Otorhinolar-yngol 2010;69:38–50.

21. Pennings R, Ho A, Brown J, et al. Analysis of Vibrant Soundbridge placement against the round window membrane in a human cadaveric temporal bone model. Otol Neurotol 2010;31(6):998–1003.

22. De S, Abajo J, Giron L, et al. Experience with the active middle ear implant in pa-tients with moderate-to-severe mixed hearing loss: indications and results. Otol Neurotol 2013;34(8):1373–9.

23. Verhaegen V, Mulder J, Cremers C, et al. Application of active middle ear im-plants in patients with severe mixed hearing loss. Otol Neurotol 2012;33(3): 297–301.

24. Schraven SP, Rak K, Shehata-Dieler W, et al. Long-term stability of the active middle-ear implant with floating-mass transducer technology: study. Otol Neuro-tol 2016;37(3):252–66.

25. Iwasaki S, Takahashi H, Kanda Y, et al. Round window application of an active middle ear implant: a comparison with hearing aid usage in Japan. Otol Neurotol 2017;38(6):e145–51.

26. Kiefer J, Arnold W, Staudenmaier R. Round window stimulation with an implant-able hearing aid (Soundbridge) combined with autogenous reconstruction of the auricle-a new approach. ORL J Otorhinolaryngol Relat Spec 2006;68(6): 378–85.

27. Frenzel H, Hanke F, Beltrame M, et al. Application of the Vibrant Soundbridge to unilateral osseous atresia cases. Laryngoscope 2009;119(1):67–74.

28. Mandalà M, Colletti L, Colletti V. Treatment of the atretic ear with round window vibrant soundbridge implantation in infants and children: electrocochleography and audiologic outcomes. Otol Neurotol 2011;32(8):1250–5.

29. Colletti L, Carner M, Veronese S, et al. The floating mass transducer for external auditory canal and middle ear malformations. Otol Neurotol 2011;32(1):108–15.

30. Colletti L, Colletti G, Colletti V. Vestibulotomy with ossiculoplasty versus round window vibroplasty procedure in children with oval window aplasia. Otol Neurotol 2014;35(5):831–7.

31. Atas A, Tutar H, Gunduz B, et al. Vibrant SoundBridge application to middle ear windows versus conventional hearing aids: a comparative study based on inter-national outcome inventory for hearing aids. Eur Arch Otorhinolaryngol 2014; 271(1):35–40.

32. Marino R, Linton N, Eikelboom RH, et al. A comparative study of hearing aids and round window application of the vibrant sound bridge (VSB) for patients with mixed or conductive hearing loss. Int J Audiol 2013;52(4):209–18.

33. Gunduz B, Atas A, Goksu N, et al. Functional outcomes of Vibrant Soundbridge applied on the middle ear windows in comparison with conventional hearing aids. Acta Otolaryngol 2012;132(12):1306–10.

34. Frenzel H, Streitberger C, Stark T, et al. The vibrant soundbridge in children and adolescents: preliminary European multicenter results. Otol Neurotol 2015;36(7): 1216–22.
35. Hüttenbrink KB, Beutner D, Bornitz M, et al. Clip vibroplasty: experimental evaluation and first clinical results. Otol Neurotol 2011;32(4):650–3.
36. Zehlicke T, Dahl R, Just T, et al. Vibroplasty involving direct coupling of the floating mass transducer to the oval window niche. J Laryngol Otol 2010; 124(7):716–9.
37. Hüttenbrink KB, Beutner D, Zahnert T. Clinical results with an active middle ear implant in the oval window. Adv Otorhinolaryngol 2010;69(69):27–31.
38. Dumon T. Vibrant soundbridge middle ear implant in otosclerosis: technique - indication. Adv Otorhinolaryngol 2007;65:320–2.
39. Kontorinis G, Lenarz T, Mojallal H, et al. Power stapes: an alternative method for treating hearing loss in osteogenesis imperfecta? Otol Neurotol 2011;32(4): 589–95.
40. Huber A, Mlynski R, Dillier N, et al. A new vibroplasty coupling technique as a treatment for conductive and mixed hearing losses: a report of 4 cases. Otol Neurotol 2012;33(4):613–7.
41. Mlynski R, Mueller J, Hagen R. Surgical approaches to position the Vibrant Soundbridge in conductive and mixed hearing loss. Operative Techniques in Otolaryngology-Head 2010;21(4):272–7.
42. Schwab B, Salcher RB, Maier H, et al. Oval window membrane vibroplasty for direct acoustic cochlear stimulation: treating severe mixed hearing loss in challenging middle ears. Otol Neurotol 2012;33(33):804–9.
43. Gostian AO, Huttenbrink KB, Luers JC, et al. Long-term results of TORP-Vibroplasty. Otol Neurotol 2015;36(6):1054–60.

Totally Implantable Active Middle Ear Implants

Michael D. Seidman, MD[a],*, Tyler A. Janz, BS[b], Jack A. Shohet, MD[c]

KEYWORDS

- The Envoy Esteem • The Carina system • Active middle ear implants
- Sensorineural hearing loss • Implantable hearing aid
- Fully implantable hearing device

KEY POINTS

- This article reviews the Esteem and Carina devices, which are active middle ear implants.
- Patients must undergo computed tomography imaging of the temporal bone and comprehensive audiometric testing to determine implant eligibility.
- Patients who cannot tolerate, are unsatisfied, or show no improvement with conventional hearing aids are candidates for the both devices.
- Clinical studies have noted either superior or similar hearing results when compared to conventional hearing aids.

INTRODUCTION

Hearing loss is the most commonly reported sensory deficit.[1] In fact, 1 out of every 5 individuals 12 years of age or older within the United States have a unilateral or bilateral hearing deficit.[2,3] To combat hearing loss, medical devices such as hearing aids are often used to amplify sound, compensating for any deficits along the auditory pathway. In the United States, an estimated 14.2% of individuals with hearing loss

Disclosures: M.D. Seidman: 7 Patents: Intellectual property; ViSalus Sciences Chief Scientific Officer/Director of Medical Advisory Board (Royalty); Acclarent Consultant; Body Language Vitamins: Founder of nutritional supplement company; Auris Medical AM 101 &111 Clinical trials for tinnitus (noncompensated research); Envoy Medical Assisting in post-market studies (noncompensated research); NIH Simulation Work/ July 2012–June 2019 (Research); MicroTransponder, Inc Vagal Nerve Stimulator Clinical Trial for tinnitus (noncompensated research). J.A. Shohet: Envoy Medical Advisory Board- Member (No Financial Interest in Company). T.A. Janz: Has nothing to disclose.
[a] Department of Otolaryngology Head and Neck Surgery, Advent Health (Celebration and South Campuses), 410 Celebration Place, Suite 305, Celebration, FL 34747, USA; [b] University of Central Florida College of Medicine, 6850 Lake Nona Boulevard, Orlando, FL 32827, USA; [c] Shohet Ear Associates, 446 Old Newport Boulevard #100, Newport Beach, Orange County, CA 92663, USA
* Corresponding author.
E-mail address: michael.seidman.md@flhosp.org

at or older than 50 years use hearing aids.[4] Hearing aids can bypass conductive middle ear disease through the amplification of sound. In addition, hearing aids can help patients with sensorineural hearing loss (SNHL) by providing amplified sound waves to the remaining hair cells within the inner ear.

Although hearing aids may improve hearing in certain patients, only approximately 30% of patients with hearing loss in the United States use hearing aids.[5] One factor for the lack of hearing aid utilization is device cost. Private and public insurance companies rarely cover hearing aids, leaving the patient to pay at costs often in the thousands of dollars.[6] Furthermore, patients may not use hearing aids due to replacement battery costs, cosmetic appearance of the hearing aid, no perceived need, or increased background noise.[7] In addition to hearing aids, other devices such as cochlear implants are often reserved for patients with severe hearing loss. Thus, although hearing aids are often used for patients with mild to moderate hearing deficiencies and cochlear implants are used for patients with severe to profound hearing deficiencies, fewer options are available for patients with moderate to severe hearing loss. One emerging option is the use of active middle ear implants. The Esteem by Envoy Medical and the Carina system by Cochlear are the only 2 totally implantable active middle ear implants currently available for patients worldwide. Although the Esteem and the Carina system have been previously discussed, recent updates regarding their use remain limited. Therefore, an updated summary of both the Esteem and Carina and their use for the treatment of hearing loss are described.

THE ESTEEM: DEVICE SUMMARY

The Esteem is a nonrechargeable battery-powered implantable hearing device consisting of a sensor, driver, and battery-powered sound processor (**Fig. 1**). The sensor is composed of a piezoelectric transducer, which is attached as a neojoint to the body of the incus. Of note, the Esteem procedure requires partial ossicular chain disruption, which allows for the sensor and driver to be cemented to their correct structures. As sound enters the external auditory canal creating movement of the tympanic membrane, malleus, and incus, the sound energy is transferred to the piezoelectric transducer, which is cemented to the incus body. The sensor transmits this signal to the battery-powered sound processor, which is implanted within the mastoid cavity. The sound processor receives, adjusts, and intensifies sound signals. Thereafter, each sound signal is sent through another piezoelectric transducer known as the "driver," which is cemented to the capitulum of the stapes. This driver translates

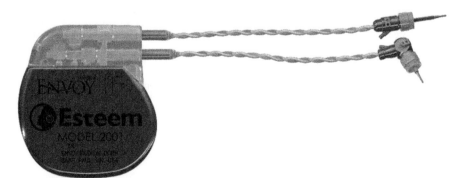

Fig. 1. The Envoy device. (*Courtesy of* Envoy Medical Corporation, White Bear Lake, MN; with permission.)

signals from the sound processor into vibrations as it vibrates the stapes against the oval window of the inner ear. Sound vibrations then proceed through the normal cochlear pathway transmitting sound signals to the brain.

THE ESTEEM: PATIENT ELIGIBILITY

Patients with bilateral moderate to severe SNHL who are 18 years of age or older are eligible to be implanted with the Esteem. Eligible patients should have had at least 30 days of experience with customized and properly fitted hearing aids. Patients should have an unaided speech discrimination score of greater than or equal to 40%. Patients additionally must have normal middle ear anatomy, normal eustachian tube function, and normal tympanic membrane function. Patients must have adequate space within the mastoid cavity to fit the Esteem, and thus all eligible patients must undergo a high-resolution computed tomography (CT) scan before the procedure. The cost for the Esteem device and procedure ranges from approximately $30,000 to $45,000. To date, most insurers have not provided reimbursement for the Esteem, and thus each patient must budget accordingly.

There are several contraindications for the implantation of the Esteem. Adult patients with chronic ear diseases such as chronic middle ear infections, cholesteatoma, mastoiditis, recurrent vertigo, Meniere disease, or fluctuating conductive hearing loss are not eligible to be implanted with the Esteem. In addition, patients who have a history of keloid formation; those with chronic wound healing issues; or those with hypersensitivities to silicone rubber, polyurethane, stainless steel, titanium, and/or gold are not recommended for implantation. As general anesthesia is required for this procedure, adequate preoperative overall health to undergo a surgical procedure is required.

THE ESTEEM: PREOPERATIVE ASSESSMENT

Patients who are eligible to be implanted with the Esteem need to be evaluated preoperatively. Surgical clearance from appropriate health care providers must be obtained before surgery. Furthermore, a surgical consent must be provided to each patient, with an adequate discussion of the risks and benefits of the Esteem procedure. Realistic expectations must be considered, and the patient must have an understanding that the Esteem may not lead to expected improvements in hearing function. Memari and colleagues'[8] prospective nonrandomized trial of 10 Esteem-implanted patients described that 2 out the 10 implanted patients did not show any hearing improvements on pure tone audiometry. Patients must be also aware of the adverse events that may happen from implanting the Esteem device. During the surgery, damage to nerves, ossicles, or other surrounding structures may occur. In addition, since the ossicular chain is being disrupted, if the device requires an explantation, a patient may experience possible hearing loss requiring additional surgery. As with any surgical procedure, risks of bleeding, infection, dizziness, vertigo, taste abnormalities, facial paralysis, and tympanic membrane perforation must be discussed with the patient.

Preoperative Computed Tomography Imaging

A preoperative CT scan must be obtained to provide the surgeon with key anatomic information to determine if the implant will fit within the mastoid cavity and provide enough space and proper angles for sensor and driver placement. Anatomic measurements or landmarks including the width of the facial recess area, the distance from the sigmoid sinus to the stapes, the sigmoid sinus anatomic location, and the distance from the tegmen to the superior ear canal need to be assessed. Of note, the distance from the sigmoid sinus to the stapes should exceed 22 mm.[9] The surgeon must additionally assess the anatomic orientation and landmarks of the temporal and parietal bones to make sure the battery-powered sound processor will fit into the temporal bone cavity.

THE ESTEEM: SURGICAL TECHNIQUE

The patient is placed in the supine, head-turned, position. General anesthesia is induced without paralytics as the facial nerve is monitored during the surgery. The patient's head is supported via a foam head rest with the operative ear facing upwards. A facial nerve monitor is placed and its proper function is verified. A microphone that is to be used during the laser Doppler vibrometry portion of the procedure is inserted into the external ear canal. The surgical field is then prepared and draped.

A postauricular incision is created and anterior and posterior flaps are made over the musculofascial layer. Once the mastoid cortex is exposed, a bony trough is drilled out posterior to the mastoid to recess the battery-powered sound processor. A wide mastoidectomy is performed. A posterior epitympanectomy is then performed exposing the head of the malleus and the incus via a wide facial recess approach (**Fig. 2**). Of note, exposure of the long process of the incus and posterior crus of the stapes must be achieved. The facial recess is then extended leading to the identification of the fibrous annulus. The chorda tympani nerve is often resected because it can impinge on the driver and may cause feedback. The incus and stapes are thereafter assessed for any abnormalities and any adhesions that may need to be removed.[9] The incus and stapes are then assessed for mobility via the use of laser Doppler vibrometry.

Laser Doppler Vibrometry

To assess for adequate ossicular movement of the incus and stapes in response to auditory stimulation, laser Doppler vibrometry is used to determine if the patient's ossicular chain will provide adequate movements to ensure a successful outcome. Before the start of the procedure, a microphone is placed within the ear canal that is used for auditory stimulation in conjunction with laser Doppler vibrometry. Once the mastoid cortex is exposed, auditory stimulation is sent through the ear canal via the microphone at the level of 100 dB across 50 different frequencies. Displacement of the ossicular chain is measured via laser Doppler vibrometry. Laser Doppler vibrometry is noted to be very accurate ($<1 \times 10^{-4}$ μm) and thus is suited to measure microscopic changes in vibratory motion as noted within the ossicular chain.[10] Extreme hypomobility of the incus or stapes is a reason to discontinue the surgery.

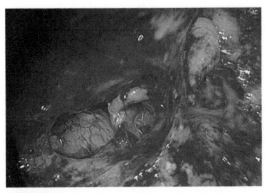

Fig. 2. Middle ear window.

Provided laser Doppler vibrometry demonstrates adequate movement of the incus and stapes, the incudostapedial joint is separated. The long process of the incus is resected using a diode laser (**Fig. 3**). Moist Gelfoam is recommended during this process to prevent exposure of adjacent structures and provide cooling within the middle ear. Once the distal segment of the long process of the incus is removed, the stapes capitulum and neck of the stapes is freed of mucosa and dried with a laser. Glass ionomeric cement (Envoycem) is then applied to the stapes capitulum and neck. The piezoelectric sensor and driver are brought onto the sterile field. They are attached to a Glasscock stabilizer to facilitate manipulation (**Fig. 4**). The sensor tip is then inserted into the epitympanum lateral to the incus body, whereas the driver tip is inserted parallel to the stapes crura lateral to the stapes capitulum[9] (**Fig. 5**). Hydroxyapatite cement (Medcem) is applied around the sensor and driver bodies to fix the transducer bodies to the mastoid. Ionomeric cement is additionally applied to both the sensor and the driver tips. The surgeon must wait for both the hydroxyapatite and ionomeric cements to harden before proceeding (**Fig. 6**). The mastoid and middle ear are then irrigated with saline and suctioned. Thereafter, the sensor and driver are tested via laser Doppler vibrometry. The sensor and driver are connected to the sound processor, and the system is activated. Laser Doppler vibrometry is then used again to measure the displacement of the incus and stapes with the Esteem system fully activated.[11] If the system is correctly functioning, the device is turned off. The surgical wound is then closed in layers, and appropriate dressings are applied.

THE ESTEEM: SURGICAL AND POSTOPERATIVE COMPLICATIONS

Given the complexity and intricacy of this surgical procedure, several surgical complications may occur. To begin with, when entering the mastoid cavity, damage to surrounding structures such as the tegmen, sigmoid sinus, and facial nerve may occur. Furthermore, before reaching the ossicular chain, damage to the ear canal or tympanic membrane may occur. Given that this procedure involves ossicular chain disruption via a laser, heat injury to surrounding structures such as the tympanic segment of the facial nerve can occur. In addition, because the incus and stapes are being manipulated, injuries such as dislocation or increased mobility to the ossicular chain bones can occur.

When applying the sensor and driver tips to the incus and stapes respectively, any slight malpositioning of these tips may lead to a device malfunction or inadequate

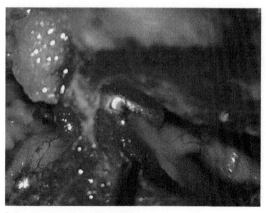

Fig. 3. Resection of the incus with a diode laser.

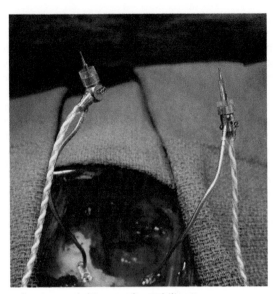

Fig. 4. Attachment of sensor and driver to the stabilizers.

response of the device. Furthermore, although cement is used to anchor these tips to their respective ossicular bones, cement fractures may occur in which additional cement may need to be applied intraoperatively. Postoperatively, if either tip from the sensor or driver becomes loose, the patient may require a revision surgery. Shohet and colleagues'[12] 5-year longitudinal study of Esteem-implanted patients noted a revision rate of 9.8%. Postoperative infections requiring explantation of the device, although possible, are extremely uncommon with rates noted to be 2.0%.[12]

Shohet and colleagues'[13] retrospective case review examined surgical complications, adverse events, and outcomes of 166 patients implanted with the Esteem. Taste disturbance was the most common adverse event occurring in 39.3% of Esteem patients. Three patients experienced a delayed facial paralysis with complete recovery. One patient (0.6%) had a traumatic injury to the facial nerve during the placement of the stabilizer bar due to a slipping of the screwdriver, which directly injured the facial nerve through the mastoidectomy defect. The facial nerve required proximal and distal

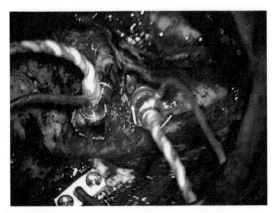

Fig. 5. Sensor and driver placement.

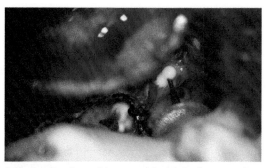

Fig. 6. Sensor and driver bodies fixated in mastoid with hydroxyapatite cement and tips cemented to incus body and stapes capitulum using glass ionomeric cement.

decompression. The patient experienced full facial nerve paralysis postoperatively with eventual recovery at 1 year to House-Brackmann II/VI. In this study, 15.7% of patients underwent revision surgery, with excess feedback occurring in 4.8% of patients, signal intermittency in 2.4% patients, and wound healing issues/excess scar tissue occurring in 4.2% of patients; 1.8% of patients underwent revision surgery after receiving minimal benefit from the device; 4.0% of patients underwent explantation of the device, with 1.8% of patients undergoing explantation for lack of perceived benefit.

THE ESTEEM: POSTOPERATIVE FOLLOW-UP

This procedure is usually performed on an outpatient basis. Patients are typically given a dose of preoperative antibiotics and another dose before discharge. They are seen 1 to 2 weeks postoperatively to check the incision site for any signs of infection, dehiscence, or hematoma. A serosanguinous effusion may occur within the middle ear that should resolve in 4 to 8 weeks. Once signs of effusion are absent, the device may be activated (usually 8 weeks postoperatively) at the first postoperative audiology appointment. Patients are then seen periodically in an effort to achieve maximal gain. Audiologists and technicians can additionally adjust the device if issues within the system arise.

THE ESTEEM: POST-IMPLANT CONTRAINDICATIONS

Previously, it was recommended that patients who were implanted with the Esteem should avoid receiving any magnetic resonance imaging (MRI). However, the Esteem device recently received conditional approval for the use of MRI. Providers should monitor for updates from the Food and Drug Administration (FDA) regarding future recommendations for the use of MRI in patients implanted with the Esteem. Furthermore, if an implanted patient undergoes any additional operations near the surgical site, the use of monopolar electrocautery should be avoided; however, if the patient is having surgery in the chest cavity or below and the ground is placed on the thigh, monopolar cautery theoretically should be safe, although bipolar cautery could be considered more prudent. Patients should notify their surgeon of the Esteem implant before undergoing any other procedures.

THE ESTEEM: BATTERY LIFE OF THE SOUND PROCESSOR

The Esteem system is powered by a nonrechargeable lithium battery. The expected battery life of the Esteem device may range from 4.5 years to 9 years depending on the frequency of use.[14] Of note, Shohet and colleagues'[12] 5-year longitudinal study of Esteem patients noted an average battery life of 4.9 years. Thus, the patient must understand that once the battery is depleted, another procedure is required to insert a new battery into the system. This battery replacement can be done under local or general anesthesia.[15] Furthermore, patients must be aware of the potential risk of a device malfunction of the battery requiring a replacement earlier than the expected battery life range.

THE ESTEEM: PROGRESSION OF HEARING LOSS

Patients may experience progression of their hearing loss leading to reduced effectiveness of the Esteem device. Otolaryngologists are discouraged from off-label implantation of the Esteem for patients with severe to profound SNHL because no perceived benefit may be noted by the patient. Patients with bilateral severe to profound SNHL should instead be considered candidates for cochlear implantation.[16] If patients who are implanted with an Esteem continue to progress with their hearing loss and are classified as severe to profound, the Esteem device may no longer be satisfactory and could be removed and replaced with a cochlear implant if they meet FDA criteria.

THE ESTEEM: CLINICAL RESULTS

In the earliest efficacy study with the original Esteem implant, Chen and colleagues[17] in 2004 implanted 7 patients, with 5 patients having a working system at the 2-month activation period. At 4 months postactivation, the functional gain of those implanted with the Esteem was 20 dB as compared with 17 dB with hearing aids. Slight improvements in speech reception thresholds (SRT) for patients implanted with the Esteem were noted as compared with each patient's best-fit hearing aid. Regarding word recognition scores (WRSs) at 50 dB, an improvement of 17% was noted after the implantation of the Esteem as compared with hearing aid conditions. Of the 7 implanted patients, 3 patients noted benefits at device activation, and 4 patients did not experience any benefit, with 3 undergoing revision surgeries in which 2 were successful.

Barbara and colleagues[18] in 2008 implanted 6 patients, with 3 patients having the device activated. The average surgical time for the procedure was 5 hours and 45 minutes (range: 3 hours and 50 minutes to 8 hours and 10 minutes). The mean (250–4000 Hz) actual hearing gains compared with the preoperative thresholds were 26 dB, 9 dB, and 11 dB.

Kraus and colleagues' prospective nonrandomized multiinstitutional phase II trial from 2008 to 2009 led to the implantation of 57 patients. Regarding SRTs, improvements compared with each patient's best-fit aid conditions were noted with the activation of the Esteem (mean best-fit aid speech threshold: 41.2 dB, 12-month post-Esteem implant: 29.4 dB [$P \le .001$]). In addition, improvements in WRSs at 50 dB were noted at 12 months postoperatively (mean best-fit aid score preimplant: 46.3%, mean 12-month post-Esteem: 68.9%). Finally, pure tone averages for post-Esteem–implanted patients improved by 27 dB (±1, 95% CI: 25–30). Of the 57 implanted patients, 6 patients were noted to have severe adverse events. Of these 6 patients, 3 revisions were completed due to fibrosis, which limited transducer functioning; 2 patients developed postoperative wound infections, which led to an explantation in one patient; and 1 patient noted delayed facial paralysis with a full functional surgical recovery.[19]

Memari and colleagues'[8] prospective nonrandomized trial led to the implantations of 10 patients with an Esteem from 2007 to 2009. The surgical time for the first 2 cases was roughly 7 hours each, whereas each of the last 2 cases took roughly 4 hours. Hearing gains were noted to be similar to conventional hearing aids (10–22 dB), although 2 out of 10 implanted patients did not show any improvements in hearing gain on pure tone audiometry; overall, patients in this study noted subjective improvements in hearing quality. Of the 10 patients, one patient experienced facial weakness without any hearing improvements and thus was explanted. Another patient underwent successful revision surgery due to excessive postoperative middle ear bone growth.

Barbara and colleagues'[20] study published in 2011 described 21 implanted patients, with 3 having mild hearing loss, 9 having moderate hearing loss (MHL), and 9 having severe hearing loss (SHL). Postoperative air conduction thresholds improved from 70 dB (preoperatively) to 48 dB for the total cohort, from 64 dB (preoperatively) to 42 dB for the MHL cohort, and from 82 dB (preoperatively) to 58 dB for the SHL cohort. The mean speech reception score at threshold levels of 60 dB (MHL) and 75 dB (SHL) increased from 42% to 79% of intelligibility for the MHL group and from 30% to 72% for the SHL group.

Gerard and colleagues'[21] study published in 2012 described 13 Esteem-implanted patients from 2008 to 2010. Postoperatively, the mean pure-tone average gain was 25 ± 11 dB. The mean word recognition score at 50 dB was $64 \pm 33\%$. Using the abbreviated profile of hearing aid benefit questionnaire, 84% of patients noted device satisfaction compared with their previously used conventional hearing aids. Five minor complications occurred, including 1 temporary facial nerve palsy, 1 secondary hearing loss, and 3 revision surgeries due to poor device function. Two patients suffered major complications requiring explantations, with both being postoperative wound infections.

Monini and colleagues'[22] retrospective study published in 2013 evaluated 15 patients who were implanted with an Esteem device. The patients were divided into 2 groups: moderate to severe SNHL (group A) and severe-to-profound SNHL (group B). Both groups were assessed without the use of any hearing aid, with the use of a conventional hearing aid, and with the Esteem implant. Significant improvements in SRTs and WRS were noted when assessing unaided values as compared with Esteem values. However, when comparing the Esteem values against conventional hearing aid values, no statistically significant differences in SRTs or WRS were noted. Esteem patients in this study noted dissatisfaction with conventional hearing aids due to several factors, including aesthetic appearance, ear canal infections, inability to wear the hearing aid at night, and interference with leisure or sporting activities. These quality of life measures were noted by patients as reasons to be implanted with the Esteem. Thus, Monini and colleagues' study noted that for patients who are dissatisfied with conventional hearing aids, the Esteem implant can offer similar improvements in hearing, with additional improvements in quality of life measures and patient compliance.

Shohet and colleagues'[12] publication enrolled 51 patients who were previously involved in their 2008 to 2009 phase II trial in a longitudinal study evaluating hearing outcomes at the 5-year mark. Forty-nine out of the 51 enrolled patients had follow-up data at the 5-year endpoint. Compared with baseline-aided conditions, SRTs improved at every annual follow-up for patients implanted with the Esteem. WRS at 50 dB were improved in 49% of patients and similarly in 41% of patients at the 5-year follow-up. WRS improved by 17% at the 5-year follow-up. Finally, the average battery life was 4.9 years. Of note, 5.8% of patients required explantation (1 being due to poor performance).

Shohet and colleagues'[13] retrospective case review in 2018 examined 166 patients with SNHL who were implanted with the Esteem from 2004 to 2015. Both the Esteem device and baseline hearing aids provided improvements in gain compared with the unaided. At both 1500 and 2000 Hz, the amount of gain was significantly greater for Esteem patients as compared with baseline-aided patients, $P<.001$. Compared with baseline-aided conditions, SRTs were significantly improved for patients implanted with the Esteem (29.9 dB vs 38.5 dB, $P<.001$). WRS at 50 dB was significantly superior in Esteem patients as compared with baseline-aided patients (65.6% vs 45.5%, $P<.001$).

THE CARINA SYSTEM: DEVICE SUMMARY

Originally developed by the Otologics company and later purchased by Cochlear Corporation, the Carina system is a fully implantable hearing prosthetic device for patients with moderate to severe SNHL or those with mixed hearing loss. The Carina system may also be used in patients with ossicular chain defects in which ossiculoplasty is not indicated or unsuccessful.[14] The Carina system consists of a microphone, rechargeable battery, magnet, sound processor, actuator, and transducer (**Fig. 7**). The transducer may be placed on the body of the incus, the stapes, the oval window, or the round window through the use of modified extensions.[23] The Carina system also includes an external charger, which charges the device through magnetic contact, as well as a remote control, which allows the user to adjust the volume and power of the device.[23] The Carina system is currently not available within the United States; however, it is available in Europe, the Middle East, and Africa.

THE CARINA SYSTEM: DEVICE OUTCOMES AND COMPLICATIONS

Compared with unaided patients, patients with the Carina system have been noted to experience a mean functional gain of 24 dB,[23] 26.4 dB,[24] or 29 dB.[25] In addition, WRS were significantly improved for Carina patients as compared with their unaided condition.[25] Compared with conventional hearing aids, no significant differences in increased functional gain or WRS were observed for patients with the Carina system implant according to Kam and colleagues.[26] However, increased perceived benefit

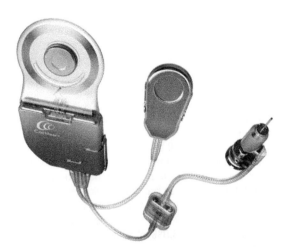

Fig. 7. The Carina system. (*Courtesy of* Cochlear Limited, © 2018. The Cochlear Carina System is not approved by the FDA for use in the United States. Cochlear and Carina are either trademarks or registered trademarks of Cochlear Limited, Sydney, Australia.)

was noted for patients implanted with the Carina system as compared with those with conventional hearing aids in Kam and colleagues' study, likely due to the "cosmetically appealing" design of the device.[26] Furthermore, Lefebvre and colleagues[27] described threshold levels for frequencies greater than 3 Hz were similar for Carina-implanted patients as compared with those with conventional hearing aids. Bruschini and colleagues[23] noted patients implanted with the Carina system expressed satisfaction with the device due to its cosmetic appealing design and ability to perform daily activities with less hindrance. Complications have been previously noted for patients implanted with the Carina system device. In 2008, Jenkins and colleagues' study of 20 patients identified ear fullness, middle ear effusion, vertigo, tinnitus, and conductive hearing loss as possible complications of the Carina system implant. In addition, Martin and colleagues'[25] study of 11 patients had 2 patients who experienced postoperative infections.

THE ESTEEM AND THE CARINA SYSTEM: SUMMARY

The Esteem is a battery-powered device designed for patients with bilateral moderate to severe SNHL who have an unaided speech discrimination score of greater than or equal to 40%. Patients who cannot tolerate, are unsatisfied, or show no improvement with conventional hearing aids are ideal candidates for the Esteem device. Furthermore, patients must undergo CT imaging of the temporal bone to identify candidates who will have a successful implantation for the Esteem. Because of the complexity of this procedure, the operation may take several hours. However, postoperative hospital stay is usually not required. Clinical studies have noted either superior or similar hearing results as compared with conventional hearing aids. Of the studies that noted similar results in comparison to conventional hearing aids, patients subjectively reported improvements in hearing as well as noted improvements in their quality of life. Although more expensive than conventional aids, the Esteem offers patients with bilateral moderate to severe SNHL another opportunity to experience improvements in hearing and lifestyle. The Carina system is a battery-powered device designed for patients with moderate to severe sensorineural hearing loss or those with mixed hearing loss. Furthermore, the Carina system offers patients the ability to charge their device externally as well as control the device via an external remote. The Esteem is currently available in the United States, whereas the Carina system is currently available only in Europe, the Middle East, and Africa.

REFERENCES

1. Hone SW, Smith RJ. Genetics of hearing impairment. Semin Neonatol 2001;6(6): 531–41.
2. Lin FR, Niparko JK, Ferrucci L. Hearing loss prevalence in the United States. Arch Intern Med 2011;171(20):1851–2.
3. Seidman MD, Ahmad N, Joshi D, et al. Age-related hearing loss and its association with reactive oxygen species and mitochondrial DNA damage. Acta Otolaryngol Suppl 2004;(552):16–24.
4. Chien W, Lin FR. Prevalence of hearing aid use among older adults in the United States. Arch Intern Med 2012;172(3):292–3.
5. Abrams H, Kihm J. An introduction to MarkeTrak IX: a new baseline for the hearing aid market. Hearing Review 2015;(22):16–21.
6. Bridges JF, Lataille AT, Buttorff C, et al. Consumer preferences for hearing aid attributes: a comparison of rating and conjoint analysis methods. Trends Amplif 2012;16(1):40–8.

7. Salonen J, Johansson R, Karjalainen S, et al. Hearing aid compliance in the elderly. B-ENT 2013;9(1):23–8.
8. Memari F, Asghari A, Daneshi A, et al. Safety and patient selection of totally implantable hearing aid surgery: Envoy system, Esteem. Eur Arch Otorhinolaryngol 2011;268(10):1421–5.
9. Marzo SJ, Sappington JM, Shohet JA. The Envoy Esteem implantable hearing system. Otolaryngol Clin North Am 2014;47(6):941–52.
10. Seidman MD, Standring RT, Ahsan S, et al. Normative data of incus and stapes displacement during middle ear surgery using laser Doppler vibrometry. Otol Neurotol 2013;34(9):1719–24.
11. Shohet JA. Esteem®: totally implantable hearing system. In: Kountakis SE, editor. Encyclopedia of otolaryngology, head and neck surgery. Berlin: Springer Berlin Heidelberg; 2013. p. 815–9.
12. Shohet JA, Kraus EM, Catalano PJ, et al. Totally implantable hearing system: Five-year hearing results. Laryngoscope 2018;128(1):210–6.
13. Shohet JA, Gende DM, Tanita CS. Totally implantable active middle ear implant: hearing and safety results in a large series. Laryngoscope 2018. [Epub ahead of print].
14. Pulcherio JO, Bittencourt AG, Burke PR, et al. Carina(R) and Esteem(R): a systematic review of fully implantable hearing devices. PLoS One 2014;9(10): e110636.
15. Bittencourt AG, Burke PR, Jardim Ide S, et al. Implantable and semi-implantable hearing AIDS: a review of history, indications, and surgery. Int Arch Otorhinolaryngol 2014;18(3):303–10.
16. Firszt JB, Holden LK, Reeder RM, et al. Cochlear implantation in adults with asymmetric hearing loss. Ear Hear 2012;33(4):521–33.
17. Chen DA, Backous DD, Arriaga MA, et al. Phase 1 clinical trial results of the Envoy System: a totally implantable middle ear device for sensorineural hearing loss. Otolaryngol Head Neck Surg 2004;131(6):904–16.
18. Barbara M, Manni V, Monini S. Totally implantable middle ear device for rehabilitation of sensorineural hearing loss: preliminary experience with the Esteem, Envoy. Acta Otolaryngol 2009;129(4):429–32.
19. Kraus EM, Shohet JA, Catalano PJ. Envoy Esteem totally implantable hearing system: phase 2 trial, 1-year hearing results. Otolaryngol Head Neck Surg 2011;145(1):100–9.
20. Barbara M, Biagini M, Monini S. The totally implantable middle ear device 'Esteem' for rehabilitation of severe sensorineural hearing loss. Acta Otolaryngol 2011;131(4):399–404.
21. Gerard JM, Thill MP, Chantrain G, et al. Esteem 2 middle ear implant: our experience. Audiol Neurootol 2012;17(4):267–74.
22. Monini S, Biagini M, Atturo F, et al. Esteem® middle ear device versus conventional hearing aids for rehabilitation of bilateral sensorineural hearing loss. Eur Arch Otorhinolaryngol 2013;270(7):2027–33.
23. Bruschini L, Berrettini S, Forli F, et al. The Carina(c) middle ear implant: surgical and functional outcomes. Eur Arch Otorhinolaryngol 2016;273(11):3631–40.
24. Bruschini L, Forli F, Passetti S, et al. Fully implantable Otologics MET Carina(™) device for the treatment of sensorineural and mixed hearing loss: audio-otological results. Acta Otolaryngol 2010;130(10):1147–53.
25. Martin C, Deveze A, Richard C, et al. European results with totally implantable carina placed on the round window: 2-year follow-up. Otol Neurotol 2009;30(8): 1196–203.

26. Kam AC, Sung JK, Yu JK, et al. Clinical evaluation of a fully implantable hearing device in six patients with mixed and sensorineural hearing loss: our experience. Clin Otolaryngol 2012;37(3):240–4.

27. Lefebvre PP, Martin C, Dubreuil C, et al. A pilot study of the safety and performance of the Otologics fully implantable hearing device: transducing sounds via the round window membrane to the inner ear. Audiol Neurootol 2009;14(3): 172–80.

Electroacoustic Stimulation

Carol Li, MD[a], Megan Kuhlmey, AuD[b], Ana H. Kim, MD[b,*]

KEYWORDS

- Electroacoustic stimulation • EAS • Hybrid cochlear implantation
- Hearing preservation

KEY POINTS

- Electric acoustic stimulation (EAS) is indicated for individuals with good low-frequency hearing and profound high-frequency hearing loss.
- EAS uses the cochlear electrode array to convey high-frequency stimuli and a hearing aid to convey low-frequency stimuli to the same ear.
- EAS shows improvement in word and sentence recognition as well as speech in noise.
- Complications associated with EAS are consistent with known risks for cochlear implantation, including loss of residual hearing.
- Progressive advancements in electrode design and atraumatic surgical techniques have resulted in improved hearing preservation and a valuable resource in the appropriate patient population.

INTRODUCTION

Electric acoustic stimulation (EAS), also known as hybrid stimulation or partial deafness cochlear implantation (CI), is indicated for individuals with intact low-frequency hearing and profound high-frequency hearing loss. Although low frequencies contribute information to aid in speech perception, speech production, environmental sound awareness, music, and emotion recognition,[1] these individuals are usually able to detect vowels, but few or no consonants, and thus have difficulty with word understanding and hearing in noise. Continuing innovations in CI have led to increased success in the preservation of residual acoustic hearing, thus allowing for the expansion of CI candidacy and the development of combined technologies in which both electric and acoustic stimulation are delivered to the implanted ear. Von Ilberg and colleagues[2] reported encouraging outcomes from the first clinical patient experience using EAS in 1999. In the EAS model, a CI electrode array (**Fig. 1**) conveys high-frequency stimuli to the implanted ear, whereas the coupled hearing aid conveys

Disclosure Statement: None.

[a] Department of Otolaryngology, Columbia University Medical Center, 180 Fort Washington Avenue, Harkness Pavilion 8th Floor, Room 864, New York, NY 10032, USA; [b] Cochlear Implant Program, Department of Otolaryngology, Columbia University Medical Center, 180 Fort Washington Avenue, Harkness Pavilion 8th Floor, Room 864, New York, NY 10032, USA
* Corresponding author.
E-mail address: ahk2166@cumc.columbia.edu

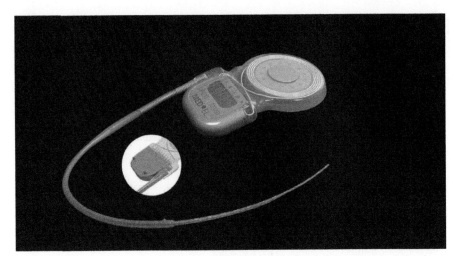

Fig. 1. Lateral wall electrode. (*Courtesy of* MED-EL Co, Durham, NC; with permission.)

low-frequency stimuli to the same ear (**Fig. 2**). Traditionally, the electrode insertion depth is confined to the basal turn of the cochlea, avoiding damage to the apical cochlear region.[3] Advances in electrode design and surgical technique have contributed to promising audiologic outcomes in clinical studies using EAS over the past

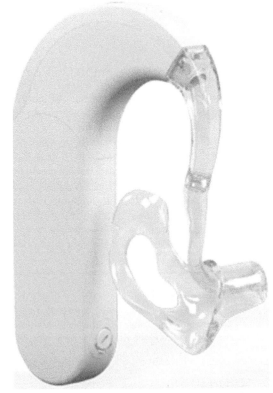

Fig. 2. EAS processor coupled with a hearing aid. (*Courtesy of* MED-EL Co, Durham, NC; with permission.)

couple of decades. This article aims to review current audiometric criteria, electrode design concepts, surgical considerations for hearing preservation, and audiologic outcomes for EAS.

AUDIOMETRIC CRITERIA FOR ELECTRIC ACOUSTIC STIMULATION

Currently, there are 2 companies that offer EAS/Hybrid options:

Cochlear America Hybrid System

Cochlear America's Hybrid system was Food and Drug Administration (FDA) approved in the United States in March 2014. FDA approved candidacy for the ear to be implanted with the Cochlear Hybrid System (Cochlear Corporation, Sydney, Australia) is summarized below and audiometric profile shown in **Fig. 3**. In brief,

- Normal hearing up to 60-dB threshold hearing loss through to 500 Hz
- Severe to profound sensorineural hearing loss in the mid to high frequencies using the average of 2 K, 3 K, and 4 K Hz, which needs to be greater than 75 dB
- Word score of 10% to 60%
- The word score of the contralateral ear should be equal or better than the ear being considered for the hybrid; however, no greater than 80%

MED-EL Electric Acoustic Stimulation System

MED-EL's EAS system (MedEl, Innsbruck, Austria) was approved in September 2016 for those meeting the following audiometric criteria (**Fig. 4**):

- Normal to moderate sensorineural hearing loss up to the mid frequencies, sloping to a severe to profound sensorineural hearing loss thereafter

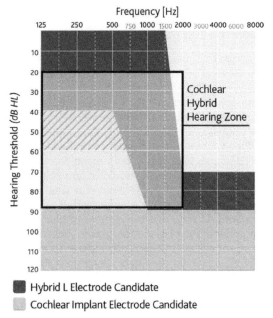

Fig. 3. Audiometric criteria with EAS indication in purple compared with traditional cochlear implant candidacy in yellow. (*Courtesy of* Cochlear Limited, Sydney, Australia; with permission.)

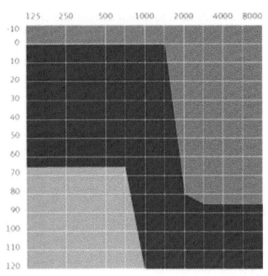

Fig. 4. MED-EL EAS audiometric profile shown in red. (*Courtesy of* MED-EL Co, Durham, NC; with permission.)

- Word score of 60% or less in the ear to be implanted

Although this criterion is inclusive of more hearing than traditional candidacy, there are considerations such as progressive hearing loss and cochlear abnormalities that need to be determined along with the audiologic criteria when considering EAS versus cochlear implant long term.

SPECIAL DEVICE DESIGN FOR ELECTRIC ACOUSTIC STIMULATION

EAS uses electrode arrays that minimize trauma during insertion and thus maximize hearing preservation. Several characteristics, such as electrode length, diameter, and degree of flexibility, contribute to atraumatic insertion. Histologic temporal bone insertion studies using flexible electrodes have demonstrated that insertion up to 1 full turn is atraumatic in the setting of correct cochleostomy techniques.[4–6] Beyond this limit, it may impart significantly increased trauma. Studies have shown that lateral wall electrodes (see **Fig. 1**) are less traumatic than precurved, perimodiolar hugging electrodes (**Fig. 5**)[7,8] because insertion occurs along the lateral wall of the scala tympani, thereby preventing trauma to the modiolus and spiral lamina.

The first application of shallow insertion electrode was reported by Gantz and Turner in 2003.[9] This Nucleus CI implant was shortened from the standard 22 mm to 6 mm and subsequently 10 mm, and the number of channels was reduced from 24 to 6. Subsequent generations of electrode design include the FlexEAS electrode (MED-EL). This electrode consists of 12 contacts and measures 20.9 mm between first and last contact. Its cross-sectional diameters vary from 0.33 × 0.49 mm at the apex to 0.8 mm at the cochleostomy site. Zigzagging of the platinum iridium wires within the silicone carrier contributes to electrode flexibility. Furthermore, the small volume and flat shape contribute to extra flexibility at the tip of the electrode. Later generations of specialized hybrid stimulation electrodes include the Flex24 (MED-EL) electrode array, measuring 24 mm in length, and the Hybrid-L electrode (Cochlear),[7,10] which has 16-mm functional length with dimensions ranging from 0.55 × 0.4 mm at the base

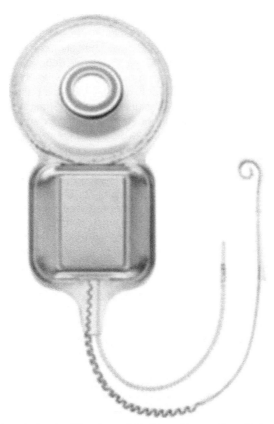

Fig. 5. Perimodiolar electrode. (*Courtesy of* Cochlear Corporation, Sydney, Australia; with permission)

to 0.35 × 0.25 mm at the apical end. More recently, Advanced Bionics have introduced their version of lateral wall electrode, Slim J, with the hope of also preserving the cochlear architecture and thereby preserving residual hearing (**Table 1**).

PRESERVATION OF RESIDUAL HEARING
Electrode Design

Many experts have examined the influence of electrode design on hearing preservation during implantation. Electrode arrays can be classified into straight and

Table 1 Summary of electrodes designed for hearing preservation			
EAS Electrode	**Year**	**Length (mm)**	**Diameter (mm)**
Cochlear nucleus	2003	6 or 10	0.2 × 0.4
MED-EL Flex[EAS] (now known as FLEX[25])	2004	20.9	0.33 × 0.49–0.8
Cochlear Hybrid-L	2006	18	0.35 × 0.25
Advanced Bionics HiFocus Slim J	2017	15	0.5–0.7

perimodiolar.[11] The first hearing preservation electrodes were straight and thus adopted a lateral wall position in lieu of the perimodiolar electrodes that were designed to lie adjacent to the modiolar wall, allowing for more spatially focused stimulation of the spiral ganglion cells. Both types of electrodes have a role depending on the patient indications. Straight electrodes are useful in patients with a variety of anatomic variations where the structure of the cochlear is not suitable for a perimodiolar electrode, such as in the case of common cavity cochlear deformity. Straight or lateral wall electrodes, such as the Slim Straight electrode (Cochlear), have demonstrated long-term low-frequency hearing preservation within 20 dB of preoperative levels in patients with usable acoustic hearing.[12] There was also significant improvement in speech understanding in quiet/noise in subjects using this electrode along with the hybrid sound processor to provide acoustic stimulation.[13] Perimodiolar electrodes aim to bring the electrode contacts closer to the neural elements of the cochlea. Studies have demonstrated a narrower spread of excitation, reduced behavioral and electrically evoked compound action potential thresholds, and wide dynamic range.[14] Perimodiolar electrodes are also applicable in a range of anatomic variations/conditions.[15] In summary, individuals with specific anatomic/medical conditions should be considered on a case-by-case basis.

Mady and colleagues[16] in 2017 compared hearing preservation outcomes using lateral wall versus perimodiolar full-length electrodes in 45 patients. At short-term follow-up, straight or lateral wall electrodes were associated with significantly better hearing preservation than perimodiolar electrodes. In multivariate regression, straight electrode use was a significant predictor of better hearing preservation. At long-term follow-up, however, electrode type was not associated with improved hearing preservation, and younger patient age was the only significant predictor of long-term hearing preservation on multivariate analysis. However, a recent meta-analysis by Santa Maria and colleagues[17] showed no disadvantage of longer electrode array length and no difference for low-frequency hearing preservation between straight versus contoured electrode arrays and electrode array type, including Cochlear's Nucleus 24-K, 24-Contour, Contour Advance, Iowa Nucleus; MED-EL's FlexEAS, FlexSoft, Combi 40+, Standard, and Custom; Advanced Bionics HiFocus Helix and Hifocus.

Perioperative Pharmacologic Interventions

Inflammation is a frequently reported reason for posttraumatic hearing loss.[18] Because of their anti-inflammatory properties, glucocorticosteroids have been and continue to be extensively examined for their effect on hearing preservation in the setting of CI. There are several animal studies supporting the use of steroids for hearing preservation.[19–22] Various preoperative, intraoperative, and postoperative regimens with topical/intravenous/oral forms have been investigated.[23–28] It is particularly difficult to penetrate the apical region of the cochlea, and it has been shown that the parenteral route is the best for covering the apical region, whereas round and/or oval window applications are best for covering the basal region.[29] Low-frequency hearing preservation has been demonstrated with the use of perioperative oral corticosteroid regimen (2-week oral corticosteroid taper beginning 3 days before surgery) in patients implanted with standard length electrodes on their first postoperative audiogram.[30] Although various studies suggest hearing preservation benefit imparted by glucocorticoids, there is no standard regimen to minimize inflammation and maximize desired outcome. The effects of steroids on wound healing in the postoperative period should also be a consideration.

Hyaluronic acid has been used as a lubricant to reduce friction trauma during electrode insertion as well as to serve as a seal around the cochleostomy to prevent perilymph leak. Antibiotic prophylaxis has also been suggested to prevent formation of bacterial biofilms at the surface of the electrode, which may lead to acute or chronic labyrinthitis.[3] The aforementioned meta-analysis by Santa Maria and colleagues in 2014[17] reported that a soft tissue seal for cochleostomy was found to be better than fibrin glue-only seal for hearing preservation. The investigators also found no benefit to postoperative oral steroids, intraoperative parenteral steroids, or preincision transtympanic steroids. They did demonstrate a beneficial effect with intraoperative topical steroids, specifically for hearing preservation at 2 kHz.

Surgical Technique

Soft surgery principles, as first described by Lehnhardt[31] in 1993, for hearing preservation during CI include avoidance of perilymph suctioning, careful manipulation around the cochleostomy, slow and delicate electrode insertion, and cochleostomy sealing. He also described a minimal cochleostomy approach, inferior and anterior to the round window. In general, there are multiple factors to consider in drilling a cochleostomy, such as acoustic trauma, presence of bone dust, and inconsistent landmarks. The round window insertion avoids these shortcomings and sets a safe morphologic landmark for the scala tympani. Kang and Kim[32] in 2013 found that patients with favorable RW anatomy who underwent round window CI electrode insertion demonstrated comparable speech perception compared with the traditional cochleostomy insertion group. Adunka and colleagues[33] in 2014 also performed a retrospective review comparing the 2 approaches in 20 patients enrolled in the EAS clinical trial. They found no statistically significant differences in postoperative outcomes for both preservation of residual hearing and unaided and aided speech perception between the 2 approaches. The true safety of approach may depend on RW orientation. Specifically, a vertical orientation may permit a fairly straight trajectory through the scala tympani, whereas a horizontal orientation makes insertion more traumatic due to deflection of the electrode by the bony cochlear hook.[33] A systematic review comparing cochleostomy versus RW approach by Havenith and colleagues[34] showed no difference in mean postoperative pure tone audiometry threshold shifts comparing both insertion techniques as well as type of electrode used (MED-EL Standard/Medium and Flex[EAS] electrode arrays). Complete low-frequency hearing preservation (defined as mean pure tone average shift at lower frequencies at 125, 250, 500, and 750 Hz, of 10 dB or less) was reported to be 0% to 40% with cochleostomy and 13% to 59% with RW approach. Complete loss of residual hearing occurred in 0% to 26% with cochleostomy and 3% to 20% with RW approach. Thus, there was no clear benefit of a specific surgical approach in this meta-analysis, but the literature is limited because there are no randomized studies with direct comparisons. Results to date suggest there might be an advantage regarding fewer patients with complete hearing loss after RW insertion. Conversely, the meta-analysis by Santa Maria and colleagues[17] report that cochleostomy is better than RW insertion in that it is more likely to yield higher rates of complete hearing preservation and trends to lower rates of partial hearing preservation. This review was different from that performed by Havenith and colleagues because they used pure tone audiometry of 250, 500, 750, 1000 ± 2000 Hz. If 2000-Hz frequency is taken into account, the cochleostomy approach has a trend toward more favorable rates of complete and partial hearing preservation.

Santa Maria and colleagues also found that mastoidectomy with posterior tympanotomy approach trended toward higher rates of complete hearing preservation compared with the suprameatal approach. Other studies found no difference.[35] Slow insertion speed showed a trend toward higher rates of hearing preservation compared with insertion speeds of less than 30 seconds because slow insertion reduces fluid forces within the cochlea.[36] Indeed, it has been shown that the slower the insertion speed, the better preservation of hearing.[37]

Systemic Inflammation

Ongoing studies are in process to define the role of inflammation in hearing preservation following CI.[38] One study in guinea pigs showed that systemic immune activation at the time of CI broadened the range of frequencies experiencing elevated thresholds after implantation. The immune activation had no significant detrimental effect on thresholds without implantation. In immune activated animals, dexamethasone treatment (20% dexamethasone phosphate adsorbed onto gelfoam and applied to the round window for 30 minutes before electrode insertion) significantly reduced threshold shifts at 2 and 8 kHz.

To date, existing literature lacks clinical evidence regarding the contribution of systemic inflammation to hearing loss or preservation after CI. There is evidence, in 2 separate longitudinal aging cohorts, that systemic inflammation is independently associated with age-related hearing loss. Using the population within the Epidemiology of Hearing Loss Study, a longitudinal cohort study of more than 1000 adults aged 48 to 92 years in Beaver Dam, Wisconsin, Nash and colleagues[39] measured markers of systemic inflammation, including serum C-reactive protein, interleukin-6, and tumor necrosis factor-α at 3 time points over a period of 22 years. The same individuals underwent audiometric testing at 2 time points to calculate a 10-year cumulative incidence of hearing impairment. Individuals less than 60 years old with high or increasing levels of serum C-reactive protein over a period of 10 years were almost 2 times more likely to develop hearing impairment. Furthermore, individuals less than 60 years of age with a higher-risk C-reactive protein profile had significantly higher pure tone averages and were more likely to experience a greater than or equal to 10-dB pure tone average progression over a period of 10 years in multivariate analyses.

ELECTRIC ACOUSTIC STIMULATION AUDIOLOGIC OUTCOMES

EAS and Hybrid systems show improvement in monosyllabic words, sentences, and speech in noise. Adunka and colleagues 2018[33] report on speech perception outcome data in the American and European trials for MED-EL EAS system, indicating that most recipients demonstrate significant improvement compared with preoperative scores on words and sentence tests.[40] Usami and colleagues[41] report improvement in monosyllabic word recognition scores from 24.1% preoperatively to 67.4% postoperatively at 1 year. Studies from Iowa University looking at the Cochlear Hybrid system indicate not only an improvement with monosyllabic words postoperatively but also overall improvement with speech understanding in noise and subjective improvement in quality of life.[42] Although the best performers used both the acoustic and the electric portions of the device, there was also improvement seen even with the electric portion alone compared with preoperative testing in all these studies.

The greatest challenges that one may face while programming EAS patients are extended appointment times due to additional counseling and testing, and integrating the acoustic and electric signals. It is recommended that one measure the unaided hearing in the audio booth before every programming session to ensure that the residual hearing has not changed. The addition of a quick threshold check will contribute to a longer appointment and greater booth utilization. The programming audiologist has to work to integrate the 2 signals for the best sound quality. More time will be spent programming to find the best crossover of acoustic signal to create the best sound quality for the patient. In addition to testing and programming, there is more coun-seling involved to manage the acoustic portion of the processor (ie, changing wax traps, ear mold impressions), which again contribute to longer appointment times.

Options with Loss of Residual Hearing

A small percentage of patients will lose residual acoustic hearing following EAS sur-gery. Gstoettner and colleagues[43] reported that 2 out of 23 patients experienced com-plete hearing loss immediately after surgery, and additional 5 patients experienced delayed hearing loss 7 to 17 months after surgery. Gantz and colleagues[44] reported complete hearing loss in 6 out of 87 patients over 3 to 24 months during the Hybrid 10 Clinical Trial. Similarly, Luetje and colleagues[45] described a delayed hearing loss at 2 and 24 months in 2 out of 13 patients. In these cases where residual hearing in the low frequencies is lost immediately or diminishes over time, individuals fall into the same scenario as conventional CI candidates with some residual hearing before surgery. Therefore, a minimum length of 18 mm is recommended for EAS in order to ensure a fully functional implant and allow for reprogramming for more electric stim-ulation for recipients who lose acoustic hearing over time.[46]

COMPLICATIONS

Complications or adverse events associated with EAS are consistent with known risks for CI. One of the most commonly reported complications is loss of residual hearing. In one multicenter clinical trial for the MED-EL EAS System, using the FLEX[25] electrode arrays, profound to total residual hearing loss occurred in 8 (11.0%) out of 73 pa-tients.[40] In long-term studies, with up to 11 years of follow-up time, Helbig and col-leagues[47] reported 22 (21.4%) cases of total hearing loss out of 103 ears implanted with different electrodes, including the MED-EL Standard, Medium, and Flex 24, and Cochlear Slim Straight. Eight of the 22 cases occurred postoperatively, whereas the other 14 cases occurred at a mean of 26 months after surgery. There were no as-sociations found between total hearing loss and electrode design or surgical approach. Other complications reported in EAS patients include type B or type C tym-panogram, conductive hearing loss, and pain at the surgical site.

Although not specifically a complication, multiple studies report the discontinuation of acoustic amplification by some EAS recipients. Some of these individuals exhibited severe to profound hearing loss in the implanted ear without sufficient hearing for the combined stimulation. Indeed, Helbig and Baumann[48] observed that acceptance of acoustic amplification occurred when individuals had residual hearing less than 75 dB in the 500-Hz frequency or below. On the other end of the spectrum, there were also individuals who rejected acoustic amplification because they retained sig-nificant amounts of residual low-frequency hearing and could combine this natural acoustic hearing with the electric stimulation.[10,49] There were also individuals who rejected acoustic stimulation due to the discomfort or inconvenience of wearing the supplementary acoustic instrument and/or external ear canal issues, such as acute external otitis media.[50]

SUMMARY

EAS was first introduced over a decade ago and has proven to be a valuable resource in the appropriate patient population. Progressive advancements in electrode design and atraumatic surgical techniques result in improved hearing preservation and consequently a demand for combined acoustic and electric stimulation.

REFERENCES

1. Gstoettner WK, Heyning P, O 'connor AF, et al. Electric acoustic stimulation of the auditory system: results of a multi-centre investigation. Acta Otolaryngol 2008; 128(9):968–75.
2. von Ilberg C, Kiefer J, Tillein J, et al. Electric-acoustic stimulation of the auditory system. New technology for severe hearing loss. ORL J Otorhinolaryngol Relat Spec 1999;61(6):334–40.
3. Kiefer J, Gstoettner W, Baumgartner W, et al. Conservation of low-frequency hearing in cochlear implantation. Acta Otolaryngol 2004;124(3):272–80.
4. Gstoettner W, Franz P, Hamzavi J, et al. Intracochlear position of cochlear implant electrodes. Acta Otolaryngol 1999;119(2):229–33.
5. Adunka O, Kiefer J. Impact of electrode insertion depth on intracochlear trauma. Otolaryngol Head Neck Surg 2006;135(3):374–82.
6. Adunka O, Kiefer J, Unkelbach MH, et al. Development and evaluation of an improved cochlear implant electrode design for electric acoustic stimulation. Laryngoscope 2004;114(7):1237–41.
7. Lenarz T, Stöver T, Buechner A, et al. Temporal bone results and hearing preservation with a new straight electrode. Audiol Neurootol 2006;11:34–41.
8. Tykocinski M, Cohen LT, Pyman BC, et al. Comparison of electrode position in the human cochlea using various perimodiolar electrode arrays. Am J Otol 2000; 21(2):205–11.
9. Gantz BJ, Turner CW. Combining acoustic and electrical hearing. Laryngoscope 2003;113(10):1726–30.
10. Lenarz T, Stöver T, Buechner A, et al. Hearing conservation surgery using the Hybrid-L electrode. Results from the first clinical trial at the Medical University of Hannover. Audiol Neurootol 2009;14(Suppl. 1):22–31.
11. Gibson P, Boyd P. Optimal electrode design: Straight versus perimodiolar. Eur Ann Otorhinolaryngol Head Neck Dis 2016;133:S63–5.
12. Jurawitz M-C, Büchner A, Harpel T, et al. Hearing preservation outcomes with different cochlear implant electrodes: nucleus® hybrid l24 and nucleus freedom Cl422. Audiol Neurootol 2014;19(5):293–309.
13. Skarzynski H, Lorens A, Matusiak M, et al. Cochlear implantation with the nucleus slim straight electrode in subjects with residual low-frequency hearing. Ear Hear 2014;35(2):e33–43.
14. Cohen LT. Practical model description of peripheral neural excitation in cochlear implant recipients: 2. Spread of the effective stimulation field (ESF), from ECAP and FEA. Hear Res 2009;247(2):100–11.
15. Bille J, Fink-Jensen V, Ovesen T. Outcome of cochlear implantation in children with cochlear malformations. Eur Arch Otorhinolaryngol 2014;2:583–9.
16. Mady LJ, Sukato DC, Fruit J, et al. Hearing preservation: does electrode choice matter? Otolaryngol Head Neck Surg 2017;157(5):837–47.
17. Santa Maria PL, Gluth MB, Yuan Y, et al. Hearing preservation surgery for cochlear implantation: a meta-analysis. Otol Neurotol 2014;35(10):e256–69.
18. Smouha EE. Surgery of the inner ear with hearing preservation: serial histological changes. Laryngoscope 2003;113(9):1439–49.
19. Chang A, Eastwood H, Sly D, et al. Factors influencing the efficacy of round window dexamethasone protection of residual hearing post-cochlear implant surgery. Hear Res 2009;255(1–2):67–72.

20. James DP, Eastwood H, Richardson RT, et al. Effects of round window dexamethasone on residual hearing in a guinea pig model of cochlear implantation. Audiol Neurootol 2008;13(2):86–96.
21. Ye Q, Kiefer J, Tillein J, et al. Intracochlear application of steroids: an experimental study in guinea pigs. Cochlear Implants Int 2004;5(Suppl. 1):17–8.
22. Ye Q, Tillein J, Hartmann R, et al. Application of a corticosteroid (Triamcinolon) protects inner ear function after surgical intervention. Ear Hear 2007;28(3):361–9.
23. Skarżyńska M, Skarżyński PH, Król B, et al. Preservation of hearing following cochlear implantation using different steroid therapy regimens: a prospective clinical study. Med Sci Monit 2018;24:2437–46.
24. Rajan GP, Kuthubutheen J, Hedne N, et al. The role of preoperative, intratympanic glucocorticoids for hearing preservation in cochlear implantation: a prospective clinical study. Laryngoscope 2012;122(1):190–5.
25. Kuthubutheen J, Joglekar S, Smith L, et al. The role of preoperative steroids for hearing preservation cochlear implantation: results of a randomized controlled trial. Audiol Neurootol 2018;22(4–5):292–302.
26. Kuthubutheen J, Coates H, Rowsell C, et al. The role of extended preoperative steroids in hearing preservation cochlear implantation. Hear Res 2014;327: 257–64.
27. Kuthubutheen J, Smith L, Hwang E, et al. Preoperative steroids for hearing preservation cochlear implantation: a review. Cochlear Implants Int 2016;17(2):63–74.
28. Cho HS, Lee KY, Choi H, et al. Dexamethasone is one of the factors minimizing the inner ear damage from electrode insertion in cochlear implantation. Audiol Neurootol 2016;21(3):178–86.
29. Maini S, Lisnichuk H, Eastwood H, et al. Targeted therapy of the inner ear. Audiol Neurootol 2009;14(6):402–10.
30. Sweeney AD, Carlson ML, Zuniga MG, et al. Impact of perioperative oral steroid use on low-frequency hearing preservation after cochlear implantation. Otol Neurotol 2015;36(9):1480–5.
31. Lehnhardt E. Intracochlear placement of cochlear implant electrodes in soft surgery technique. HNO 1993;41(7):356–9.
32. Kang BJ, Kim AH. Comparison of cochlear implant performance after round window electrode insertion compared with traditional cochleostomy. Otolaryngol Head Neck Surg 2013;48(5):822–6.
33. Adunka OF, Dillon MT, Adunka MC, et al. Cochleostomy versus round window insertions: Influence on functional outcomes in electric-acoustic stimulation of the auditory system. Otol Neurotol 2014;35(4):613–8.
34. Havenith S, Lammers MJW, Tange RA, et al. Hearing preservation surgery: Cochleostomy or round window approach? A systematic review. Otol Neurotol 2013; 34(4):667–74.
35. Bruijnzeel H, Draaisma K, van Grootel R, et al. Systematic review on surgical outcomes and hearing preservation for cochlear implantation in children and adults. Otolaryngol Head Neck Surg 2016;154(4):586–96.
36. Kontorinis G, Lenarz T, Stöver T, et al. Impact of the insertion speed of cochlear implant electrodes on the insertion forces. Otol Neurotol 2011;32(4):565–70.
37. Rajan GP, Kontorinis G, Kuthubutheen J. The effects of insertion speed on inner ear function during cochlear implantation: a comparison study. Audiol Neurootol 2012;18(1):17–22.
38. Verschuur C, Causon A, Green K, et al. The role of the immune system in hearing preservation after cochlear implantation. Cochlear Implants Int 2015;16(sup1): S40–2.

39. Nash SD, Cruickshanks KJ, Zhan W, et al. Long-term assessment of systemic inflammation and the cumulative incidence of age-related hearing impairment in the epidemiology of hearing loss study. J Gerontol A Biol Sci Med Sci 2014; 69(2):207–14.

40. Pillsbury H, Dillion M, Buchman C, et al. Mulitcenter clinical trial with an electro-acoustic stimulation (EAS) system in adults: final outcomes. Otol Neurotol 2018; 39:299–305.

41. Usami S, Moteki H, Tsukada K, et al. Hearing preservation and clinical outcome of 32 consecutive electric acoustic stimulation (EAS) surgeries. Acta Otolaryngol 2014;134(7):717–27.

42. Gantz B, Turner C, Gfeller K, et al. Preservation of hearing in cochlear implant surgery: advantages of combined electrical and acoustical speech processing. Laryngoscope 2005;115:796–802.

43. Gstoettner WK, Heibig S, Maier N, et al. Ipsilateral electric acoustic stimulation of the auditory system: results of long-term hearing preservation. Audiol Neurootol 2006;11(Suppl 1):49–56.

44. Gantz BJ, Hansen MR, Turner CW, et al. Hybrid 10 clinical trial: preliminary results. Audiol Neurootol 2009;14(Supple 1):32–8.

45. Luetje CM, Thedinger BS, Buckler LR, et al. Hybrid cochlear implantation: clinical results and critical review in 13 cases. Otol Neurotol 2007;28(4):473–8.

46. Helbig S, Helbig M, Rader T, et al. Cochlear reimplantation after surgery for electric-acoustic stimulation. ORL J Otorhinolaryngol Relat Spec 2009;71(3): 172–8.

47. Helbig S, Adel Y, Rader T, et al. Long-term hearing preservation outcomes after cochlear implantation for electric-acoustic stimulation. Otol Neurotol 2016;37(9): e353–9.

48. Helbig S, Baumann U. Acceptance and fitting of the DUET device - a combined speech processor for electric acoustic stimulation. Adv Otorhinolaryngol 2010; 67:81–7.

49. Skarzynski H, Lorens A, Piotrowska A, et al. Preservation of low frequency hearing in partial deafness cochlear implantation (PDCI) using the round window surgical approach. Acta Otolaryngol 2007;127(1):41–8.

50. Helbig S, Van de Heyning P, Kiefer J, et al. Combined electric acoustic stimulation with the PULSARCI(100) implant system using the FLEX(EAS) electrode array. Acta Otolaryngol 2011;131(6):585–95.

Special Populations in Implantable Auditory Devices: Pediatric

Jennifer R. White, MD[a], Diego A. Preciado, MD, PhD[b],
Brian K. Reilly, MD[b],*

KEYWORDS

- Pediatric • Implantable auditory devices • Bone-conduction device
- Cochlear implant

KEY POINTS

- There is substantial support for performing the osseointegrated bone-conduction devices in patients as young as 3 years old, with the critical factors being bone density and skull thickness.
- Studies have found that patients with severe to profound sensorineural hearing loss (SNHL) receiving cochlear implantation (CI) when younger than 12 months are able to reach their full hearing potential without having to play "catch up" to their peers.
- Confirmation of CI placement is usually achieved with a combination of intraoperative evoked compound action potential and radiologic testing with plain radiographs.
- The auditory results of auditory brainstem implants vary widely; many patients having only improved lip-reading scores and sound awareness.

INTRODUCTION

Hearing loss rehabilitation in the pediatric population is imperative to ensure the proper development of language, speech, and social skills. The 1-3-6 rule (screen for hearing loss by age 1 month, complete a diagnostic audiologic evaluation by age 3 months, and enroll in appropriate early intervention services by age 6 months) provides a timeline for diagnosis and intervention and can help assist which modality of hearing rehabilitation is best suited for the child.[1] Earlier referral and intervention is critical to prevent auditory deprivation during this time-sensitive period of

Disclosure Statement: The authors have nothing to disclose.
[a] Department of Otolaryngology, Medstar Georgetown University Hospital, 3800 Reservoir Road Northwest, Washington, DC 20007, USA; [b] Division of Pediatric Otolaryngology, Children's National Health System, George Washington University School of Medicine, 111 Michigan Avenue Northwest, Washington, DC 20010, USA
* Corresponding author.
E-mail address: breilly@cnmc.org

Otolaryngol Clin N Am 52 (2019) 323–330
https://doi.org/10.1016/j.otc.2018.11.015
0030-6665/19/© 2018 Elsevier Inc. All rights reserved.

development. The following discussion outlines rehabilitation options for these patients, with specific focus on implantable auditory devices.[2]

OSSEOINTEGRATED BONE-CONDUCTION DEVICES

Osseointegrated bone-conduction hearing devices (OBCD) were first trialed in 1977 in adults in Sweden and have since been a treatment option for hearing loss in more than 30,000 patients worldwide.[3] The use in children was first reported in 1983.[4] The indications and candidacy guidelines for OBCDs have expanded since their initial use and now include treatment of unilateral or bilateral conductive hearing loss (CHL) (eg, in children with aural atresia, chronic otitis media, ossicular abnormalities), unilateral or bilateral mixed hearing loss, those with the inability to use a traditional air-conduction hearing aid or a contralateral routing of the signal (CROS) hearing aid, as well as profound unilateral sensorineural hearing loss (SNHL) in the setting of normal-hearing contralateral ear, also known as single-sided deafness (SSD). The Food and Drug Administration (FDA) approved the use of OBCDs in adults in 1996 and in children older than 5 years in 1999. In 2002, the FDA approved its use in SSD. There is no current FDA approval for use in children younger than 5 years, although these children can use a temporary external softband with the OBCD device attached to it until they are old enough to undergo surgery.[5] Although the FDA recommends performing the surgery in patients 5 years and older, there is substantial support for performing the BAHA surgery in patients as young as 3 years old in the medical literature. In fact, the surgery has been done successfully in children as young as 18 months old, and the European Union has approved percutaneous OBCD implants for patients 3 years old.

The OBCD is a surgically implantable system that was created to take advantage of the high speed (low impedance) at which sound can travel through bone. It specifically conducts amplified sound directly and immediately to the cochlea from its abutment placed in the parietal bone, as seen in **Fig. 1**.[3] The procedure for the implant is usually performed on an outpatient basis. Both single- and 2-stage procedures are available depending on the patient age, skull thickness, and surgeon's preference. In the pediatric population, 2-stage surgery is performed to allow proper time for osseointegration of the OBCD abutment when there is concern about bone density or skull thickness.[6] The main message regarding pediatric OBCD implantation is understanding the issues regarding skull thickness that may lead to implantation of 3-mm rather than 4-mm BAHA (Cochlear Ltd, Molnkycke, Sweden) or Ponto (Oticon Medical, Somerset, New Jersey) implants, and implantation of a "sleeper" in case the first one extrudes; or implantation of the Sophono "upside down" to avoid drilling wells that project onto the dura mater.

One of the main disadvantages to the percutaneous OBCD is soft tissue reaction at the site of the abutment, which can range from mild erythema to complete skin overgrowth requiring surgical revision, as seen in **Fig. 2**. As such, there is a high degree of abutment maintenance and skin hygiene that can be required to maintain the tissue health around the device. In some instances, soft tissue granulation requires temporary cessation in use of the device while the patient is being treated with steroid creams and antibiotics. Children, in particular, must be encouraged not to play with, or "wiggle" their percutaneous abutment, as that can cause failure of osseointegration and subsequent implant extrusion. The release of the BAHA Attract (Cochlear, Ltd, Mölnlycke, Sweden) and Sophono (Sophono Inc, Boulder, CO) systems has greatly improved this soft tissue issue. These OBCD devices are composed of a completely

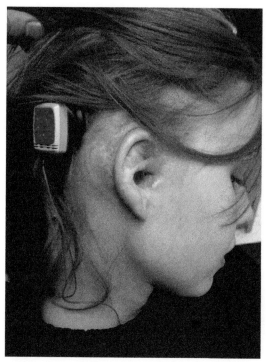

Fig. 1. Pediatric patient with an OBCD (Baha Attract). (*Courtesy of* Cochlear Americas, Centennial, CO © 2018. with permission.)

subcutaneous magnet that inserts in the osseointegrated implant rather than a percutaneous abutment.[7] All devices, whether percutaneous or transcutaneous (magnetic) involve an external component.

The decision to proceed with an OBCD typically depends on hearing thresholds using age-appropriate hearing tests, subjective trial of a bone conductor or softband device, and comfort levels of the child and guardians after counseling.[5] Currently, the external device on a softband, available from all 3 OBCD companies (BAHA, Sophono, and Ponto) is the most appropriate means to provide aural rehabilitation to children younger than 3. The use of the OBCD on a soft headband is the gold standard for audiological preoperative assessment in children. A challenge in the management of older children is peer pressure and self-esteem regarding the appearance of the test bands. This can result in poor compliance despite good audiological outcomes. Similarly, those children with learning difficulties may have problems accepting the softband.[8]

Although many OBCD candidates have normal hearing in one ear, developmental, educational, and social implications of unilateral hearing loss are well documented, making early identification and intervention a vital part of ensuring the child's success. As many as 22% to 35% of children with unilateral hearing loss repeat at least one school grade and up to 40% require educational assistance.[9] Numerous studies have outlined beneficial outcomes with OBCD, encompassing improved quality of life, improved hearing outcomes, and compliance with device usage.[10] The use of a single implantable device may be a better option for patients unwilling or unable to wear multiple hearing aids or removable devices. This is particularly important in pediatric populations, in which compliance is a concern.[11] Purcell and colleagues[12]

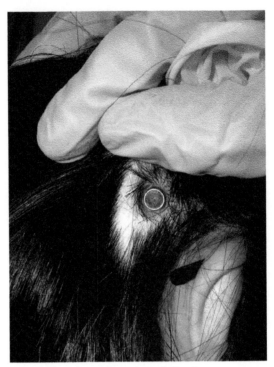

Fig. 2. Local inflammation and granulation tissue following percutaneous osseointegrated bone-conduction implantation in a pediatric patient.

looked at a cohort of pediatric patients and found that the retention rates for CROS and behind-the-ear devices were 69% and 47% regardless of patient age. The most common reason for cessation was discomfort and lack of benefit. On the contrary, McDermott and colleagues[13] reported daily use in 97% of a cohort of patients with an OBCD. OBCDs have also been found to have improved hearing in noise when compared with traditional CROS hearing aids, a benefit that can be particularly useful in the classroom.[11] In terms of patient satisfaction, the literature has shown an increase in satisfaction surveys, including the Glasgow Children's Benefit Inventory and SSD Questionnaire after implantation with OBCD.[14]

MIDDLE EAR IMPLANTS

Initially introduced in the 1990s, the Vibrant Soundbridge (VSB; MED-EL Corporation, Innsbruck, Austria) is a middle ear implant that was initially developed for patients with SNHL.[15] However, the indications have since been expanded and now encompass patients with mixed and CHL. This provides an alternative hearing rehabilitation option for patients with congenital aural atresia, microtia, or extensive middle ear malformation in whom reconstruction surgery is not likely to be sufficient or stable.[16] Although not FDA approved in children, in unique cases, patients younger than 18 years have been implanted, with the first reported implantation in a child being performed in June 2009.[15]

The principle behind the middle ear implant is based on the direct drive of the ossicular chain using mechanical vibrations, which are relayed by an implanted transducer. Implantation of the device requires an operation under general anes-thesia, in which the vibrating ossicular prosthesis (VORP) is implanted subcutane-ously. The floating mass transducer (FMT) is then placed on the round window, oval window, mobile stapes remnants, or on the long process of the incus. The audio processor is held in place externally with a magnet, and this receives audio signals by a microphone system, which then sends them to the VORP. The VORP then con-verts this sound into mechanical vibrations, which are carried out by the FMT. Fre-quency information up to 8 kHz can be delivered via this system. In experienced hands, this is a challenging but relatively safe operation, which requires a surgical approach similar to cochlear implants (CIs) through the facial recess. It is therefore not without risk of potential damage to the facial nerve, chorda tympani, or middle ear structures.[17]

The benefit of this system over bone-conduction devices is its ability to treat unilateral hearing loss without involving the contralateral ear, which may aid in binaural hearing and sound localization. Audiologic outcomes in the pediatric population have been promising. Frenzel and colleagues[16] reported results from a group of 19 pediatric patients from 5 to 17 years of age and found a significant improvement in speech discrimination after 6 months in all age groups. In addition, Leinung and colleagues[15] reported parent-perceived outcomes of VSB for children with unilateral congenital aural atresia as compared with bone-conduction devices and found significant improvement in acceptance by the child, listening effort, handling, behavior, and qual-ity of life. They also found a difference in daily use of 10 hours for VSB as compared with 2 hours for bone-conducting devices.

COCHLEAR IMPLANTS

An estimated 1 of every 1000 neonates in the United States is born with profound bilateral sensorineural loss (SNHL), which may be due to a multitude of etiologies, including genetic, pharmacologic, toxic, and metabolic factors. The damage lies in the sensory hair cells of the Organ of Corti. CIs provide a means to bypass this and directly stimulate the cochlear nerve ganglia, thereby transmitting electrical signals to the brain, which are ultimately perceived as sound. CI has allowed these children with severe to profound SNHL to gain intelligible speech and spoken lan-guage skills early in their development that rivals that of their normally hearing peers.[18]

Approximately 40,000 CIs have been performed on pediatric patients as of December 2012.[19] Audiologic threshold criteria for candidacy are as follows: greater than 90 dB hearing loss (HL) (3-frequency pure-tone average) for children ages 12 to 23 months and greater than 70 dB HL (Cochlear) or greater than 90 dB HL (Advanced Bionics, Valencia, CA, or MED-EL, Durham, NC) for children older than 2 years. In addition to poor scores on age-appropriate speech recogni-tion tests, patients must also show limited improvement with binaural hearing aids. Recent studies indicate that lower audiologic thresholds (80 dB HL) should be considered in the candidacy criteria for children as well.[2] In addition, CIs are currently FDA approved only for children older than 12 months. However, studies have found that patients implanted when younger than 12 months are able to reach their full potential without having to play "catch up" to their peers. Kim and col-leagues[18] found that infants receiving a cochlear implant had no more general sur-gical complications in the immediate postoperative period as compared with older children. However, they did have a significantly greater total operative time, length of stay, and readmission rate.

The use of preoperative imaging in the pediatric population is imperative given that the rate of anatomic abnormalities in pediatric CI candidates with congenital hearing loss is approximately 20%. The best imaging modality is still debated, and the risk-benefit ratio should be considered for both computed tomography (CT) and MRI. Most anomalies can be identified with either imaging modality. A hypoplastic acoustic nerve is better visualized with an MRI; however, most of the time this is accompanied by a narrowed internal auditory canal or cochlear or vestibular dysplasia, which is better appreciated on CT. MRI scans often require sedation in the pediatric population, but there is also an inherent risk of radiation exposure that comes with CT scans.[20]

The high rate of anatomic abnormalities in this patient population also puts the patients at risk for electrode array misplacement, such as tip fold-over, kinking, overinsertion or underinsertion, or looping, which can affect the audiologic outcomes. Confirmation of placement is usually achieved with a combination of intraoperative evoked compound action potential (ECAP) and radiologic testing with plain radiographs. Some studies argue that imaging is indicated only in cases of abnormal ECAP or suspicion of misplacement. Cosetti and colleagues,[19] however, found the rate of misplacement to be 1.8% in a cohort of 277 pediatric patients with CI with normal cochleovestibular anatomy, and 2 of the 5 children with abnormal radiographs had normal neural response telemetry (NRT) and no concern intraoperatively for misplacement. The conclusion was to advocate for intraoperative radiographs in all cases, irrespective of NRT.

AUDITORY BRAINSTEM IMPLANTS

The auditory brainstem implant (ABI) is a surgically implanted prosthetic device that provides an auditory rehabilitation option for deaf patients who do not benefit from a CI. It was originally developed at the House Ear Institute for patients with neurofibromatosis type 2 (NF2), given their propensity to develop bilateral vestibular schwannomas leading to eventual profound hearing loss. It was FDA approved in 2000 for patients with NF2 who were 12 years or older.[21] The implant bypasses the damaged or absent cochlea and auditory nerve and is placed at the cochlea nucleus in the brainstem to provide direct stimulation.

The indications for ABI have expanded since its initial development to include non-NF2 adults and children who have a severely hypoplastic or absent cochlea, a small or absent auditory nerve, or injury or scarring of the inner ear or auditory nerve secondary to meningitis, trauma, or tumor.[22] The use of ABI in children without NF2 has increased throughout the world. The auditory results vary widely, with many patients having only improved lip-reading scores and sound awareness (Kaplan, Fort Lauderdale, FL). However, overall patients without NF2 have been found to have better outcomes than patients with NF2. One theory for this is that tumor resection in patients with NF2 may affect correct placement of the electrodes.[21]

Until 2012, no ABIs had been performed on non-NF2 pediatric patients in the United States. The FDA has since approved trials at Massachusetts Eye and Ear Infirmary, University of North Carolina-Chapel Hill, House Ear Institute, and New York University to perform ABI surgeries on children without NF2 with congenital and acquired malformations of the cochlea and auditory nerve.[22] Preliminary 1-year data published by the House Institute have been promising, with 4 of the 5 patients with speech detection thresholds of 30 to 35 dB HL. The surgery is not without complications; however, no patients have had long-term negative sequela. Some perioperative complications encountered include cerebrospinal fluid leak, vestibular symptoms, and postoperative emesis[21] (**Box 1**).

Box 1
Conclusion

- Hearing loss rehabilitation in the pediatric population is imperative to ensure the proper development of language, speech, and social skills.

- Osseointegrated bone-conduction devices are approved by the Food and Drug Administration (FDA) for children older than 5 years. Osseointegrated bone-conduction hearing devices are a suitable option for patients unable to wear traditional hearing aids, such as children with microtia, or those who do not tolerate them.

- Middle ear implants have been implanted in patients younger than 18 years since 2009. The advantage of this system over bone-conduction devices is the ability to treat unilateral hearing loss without affecting the contralateral ear. This may improve sound localization and binaural hearing for patients.

- Cochlear implants are FDA approved for children older than 12 months, although studies looking at earlier implantation have found that these children are able to reach their full potential without having to "catch up" to their peers without risk of increased complication rate.

- Preoperative imaging before cochlear implantation is important to rule out anatomic abnormalities, with the preferred imaging modality being MRI, computed tomography, or both. The high rate of anatomic abnormalities within this patient population also puts patients at risk for electrode array misplacement. Proper positioning can be confirmed with both intraoperative ECAP and plain radiographs.

- Auditory brainstem implants may be an auditory rehabilitation option for deaf patients who do not benefit from a cochlear implant. The indications have expanded over the years to now include patients without neurofibromatosis type 2 (NF2) who have severely hypoplastic or absent cochlea, a small or absent auditory nerve, or injury or scarring of the inner ear or auditory nerve secondary to meningitis, trauma, or tumor. Preliminary FDA-approved trials in the United States on children without NF2 are under way, and the results thus far are promising.

REFERENCES

1. Muse C, Harrison J, Yoshinaga-Itano C, et al. Supplement to the JCIH 2007 position statement: principles and guidelines for early intervention after confirmation that a child is deaf or hard of hearing. Pediatrics 2013;131(4):e1324–49.

2. de Kleijn JL, van Kalmthout LWM, van der Vossen MJB, et al. Identification of pure-tone audiologic thresholds for pediatric cochlear implant candidacy: a systematic review. JAMA Otolaryngol Head Neck Surg 2018;144(7):630–8.

3. Christensen L, Richter GT, Dornhoffer JL. Update on bone-anchored hearing aids in pediatric patients with profound unilateral sensorineural hearing loss. Arch Otolaryngol Head Neck Surg 2010;136(2):175.

4. Kraai T, Brown C, Neeff M, et al. Complications of bone-anchored hearing aids in pediatric patients. Int J Pediatr Otorhinolaryngol 2011;75(6):749–53.

5. Kubala ME, Cox MD, Nelson KL, et al. Influence of behavior on complications of osseointegrated bone conduction devices in children. Otol Neurotol 2017;38(4):535–9.

6. Saliba I, Froehlich P, Bouhabel S. One-stage vs. two-stage BAHA implantation in a pediatric population. Int J Pediatr Otorhinolaryngol 2012;76(12):1814–8.

7. Cedars E, Chan D, Lao A, et al. Conversion of traditional osseointegrated bone-anchored hearing aids to the Baha® attract in four pediatric patients. Int J Pediatr Otorhinolaryngol 2016;91:37–42.

8. Mcdermott AL, Sheehan P. Bone anchored hearing aids in children. Curr Opin Otolaryngol Head Neck Surg 2009;17(6):488–93.

9. Lieu JE. Speech-language and educational consequences of unilateral hearing loss in children. Arch Otolaryngol Head Neck Surg 2004;130(5):524.

10. Amonoo-Kuofi K, Kelly A, Neeff M, et al. Experience of bone-anchored hearing aid implantation in children younger than 5 years of age. Int J Pediatr Otorhinolaryngol 2015;79(4):474–80.

11. Dornhoffer JR, Dornhoffer JL. Pediatric unilateral sensorineural hearing loss. Curr Opin Otolaryngol Head Neck Surg 2016;24(6):522–8.

12. Purcell PL, Jones-Goodrich R, Wisneski M, et al. Hearing devices for children with unilateral hearing loss: patient- and parent-reported perspectives. Int J Pediatr Otorhinolaryngol 2016;90:43–8.

13. McDermott AL, Williams J, Kuo M, et al. The Birmingham pediatric bone-anchored hearing aid program: a 15-year experience. Otol Neurotol 2009; 30(2):178–83.

14. Doshi J, Banga R, Child A, et al. Quality-of-life outcomes after bone-anchored hearing device surgery in children with single-sided sensorineural deafness. Otol Neurotol 2013;34(1):100–3.

15. Leinung M, Zaretsky E, Lange BP, et al. Vibrant Soundbridge® in preschool children with unilateral aural atresia: acceptance and benefit. Eur Arch Otorhinolaryngol 2016;274(1):159–65.

16. Frenzel H, Sprinzl G, Streitberger C, et al. The Vibrant Soundbridge in children and adolescents: preliminary European multicenter results. Otol Neurotol 2015; 36(7):1216–22.

17. Bruchhage KL, Leichtle A, Schönweiler R, et al. Systematic review to evaluate the safety, efficacy and economical outcomes of the Vibrant Soundbridge for the treatment of sensorineural hearing loss. Eur Arch Otorhinolaryngol 2016;274(4): 1797–806.

18. Kim Y, Patel VA, Isildak H, et al. An analysis of safety and adverse events following cochlear implantation in children under 12 months of age. Otol Neurotol 2017;38(10):1426–32.

19. Anne S, Juarez JM, Shaffer A, et al. Utility of intraoperative and postoperative radiographs in pediatric cochlear implant surgery. Int J Pediatr Otorhinolaryngol 2017;99:44–8.

20. Tamplen M, Schwalje A, Lustig L, et al. Utility of preoperative computed tomography and magnetic resonance imaging in adult and pediatric cochlear implant candidates. Laryngoscope 2015;126(6):1440–5.

21. Wilkinson EP, Eisenberg LS, Krieger MD, et al. Initial results of a safety and feasibility study of auditory brainstem implantation in congenitally deaf children. Otol Neurotol 2017;38(2):212–20.

22. Kaplan AB, Kozin ED, Puram SV, et al. Auditory brainstem implant candidacy in the united states in children 0-17 years old. Int J Pediatr Otorhinolaryngol 2015; 79(3):310–5.

Special Populations in Implantable Auditory Devices: Geriatric

Selena E. Briggs, MD, PhD, MBA, MAUML[a,b],*

KEYWORDS

- Geriatric • Elderly • Hearing loss • Implantable hearing aid • Implantable
- Bone conduction hearing aid

KEY POINTS

- Hearing loss is one of the major chronic illnesses among the elderly.
- Hearing loss is associated with significant impact on patient psychological, cognitive, and social well-being in the elderly population.
- In addition to conventional hearing aids, implantable hearing devices are an exceptional option for aural rehabilitation in the elderly population.
- Counseling is required to establish realistic expectations.
- Rehabilitation is required to optimize results.

INTRODUCTION

Hearing loss is one of the most common conditions impacting the aging population. In the United States, hearing loss is among the top 3 most common condition affecting the aging population and is the most common communication disorder affecting the geriatric population.[1,2] Within the population over the age of 65 years, at least 1 in 3 individuals are affected with hearing loss; this number increases significantly with age, such that more than 50% of individuals over the age of 80 have some degree of hearing loss.[2–4] By 2050, it is expected that the population of individuals within this demographic will double worldwide owing to a significant increase in human lifespan with improved medical care; thus, a corresponding increase in the rates of hearing loss encountered and associated comorbidities.[5] Presbycusis or age-related hearing loss is the etiologic factor in the vast majority of geriatric patients with hearing

[a] Department of Otolaryngology, MedStar Washington Hospital Center, 106 Irving Street NW, Suite 2700 North, Washington, DC 20010; [b] Department of Otolaryngology, MedStar Georgetown University Medical Center, Gorman Building, 1st Floor, 3800 Reservoir Road NW, Washington, DC 20007
* 106 Irving Street NW, Suite 2700 North, Washington, DC 20010.
E-mail address: Heman.oto@gmail.com

Otolaryngol Clin N Am 52 (2019) 331–339
https://doi.org/10.1016/j.otc.2018.11.009
0030-6665/19/© 2018 Elsevier Inc. All rights reserved.

loss. However, the etiology of hearing loss within the geriatric population can be multi-factorial in nature, including but not limited to noise exposure, trauma, infection, otosclerosis, or cholesteatoma, leading to a mixed/conductive component to hearing loss within this population.

IMPACT OF HEARING LOSS IN THE GERIATRIC POPULATION

Hearing loss can have a significant impact on individuals within the geriatric population and the understanding of this impact is ever increasing in health care. Hearing loss in the geriatric population has been associated with overall decrease in quality of life.[6-8] Geriatric patients often experience social isolation and anxiety in social situations associated with the frustration and embarrassment of their communication challenges.[9,10] This has been demonstrated to progress to decreased autonomy, loneliness and depression, significantly impacting their activity level and social interconnectivity.[10-18] Hearing loss in the geriatric population also has a significant impaction on cognition and mentation.

The association between dementia and age-related hearing loss has been described for decades within the literature with our understanding of its impact evolving significantly within the past decade. A significant correlation between hearing impairment and progression of dementia was reported within the literature starting in the mid 1980s.[11,19,20] Additionally, age-related hearing loss was noted to be associated with global functional decline.[9,21,22] A direct positive correlation between degree of hearing loss and cognitive decline has been noted on cognitive testing in numerous reports in the literature.[11,23-28] Quantitatively in recent literature, the impact of the degree of hearing was associated with cognitive decline in individuals free of prevalent dementia or mild cognitive impairment. A 25-dB hearing loss was noted to produce a decline equivalent to an age difference of 6.8 years on test of executive function.[29,30] Remarkably, adequate aural rehabilitation has been demonstrated to mitigate the negative impact of hearing loss in the geriatric population.

AURAL REHABILITATION DECREASES THE IMPACT OF HEARING LOSS IN GERIATRIC PATIENTS

Hearing loss has a wide-reaching impact on the lives of geriatric patients. Aural rehabilitation has been found to eliminate or diminish the deleterious effect of hearing loss in the aging population. Cochlear implantation and hearing aid use have been demonstrated to improve overall quality of life in the geriatric population.[6,31,32] The psychosocial impact of hearing loss has also been noted to be positively impacted by adequate aural rehabilitation. With augmentation of hearing in the geriatric population, anxiety, social isolation, depression, and stress have been demonstrated to decrease significantly.[17-19,32] The influence of hearing loss on cognition is also impacted with aural rehabilitation. With use of cochlear implants and hearing aids, cognitive decline has been noted to be independently associated with hearing loss and impact the severity of cognitive decline or dementia.[33]

Options for Aural Rehabilitation in the Geriatric Population

The determination of aural rehabilitative strategy is largely predicated on the character and severity of the patient's hearing loss. For individuals with early signs of hearing loss or borderline findings noted on audiometric evaluation, environmental optimization may be used with a focus on optimizing the patient's auditory milieu including minimizing ambient noise during conversation (eg, television and music) and selecting more favorable seating to allow face to face conversation. Simple amplification devices may be used in early stages of hearing loss to augment sound intensity in conjunction with these optimization measures.

Conventional hearing aids remain the mainstay of treatment for geriatric patients with hearing loss. Hearing aids are typically indicated for individuals with hearing thresholds of 40 dB or greater within the speech frequencies with adequate speech understanding (typically speech discrimination of >50% to 60%). Hearing aid use is largely independent of the character of hearing loss (amiable to unilateral or bilateral hearing loss; sensorineural, mixed, or conductive hearing loss). For geriatric patients with severe to profound bilateral hearing loss, cochlear implantation may be an option. Cochlear implantation is recommended for patients who do not derive benefit from hearing aid use and meet certain criteria for speech discrimination testing (ie, score ≤50% on sentence recognition testing in their worse hearing ear and ≤60% in the bilateral best aided conditions). These criteria for implantation particularly within the geriatric population are ever evolving and broadening to encompass a greater degree of residual hearing. Within the geriatric population, the procedure is typically performed in the outpatient setting unless precluded by medical comorbidities and is well-tolerated, with low surgical morbidity and high rates of success.[34–40] Interestingly, unlike hearing aids, cochlear implantation is covered by most health care plans. In addition to cochlear implantation, implantable auditory devices are gaining popularity in the treatment of hearing loss within the geriatric population.

IMPLANTABLE HEARING DEVICES IN THE GERIATRIC POPULATION

Implantable hearing devices (IHDs) are increasing in popularity within the geriatric population as an option for aural rehabilitation. Unlike cochlear implants, which convert external sound wave stimuli into an electrical signal for direct stimulation of the cochlea for aural rehabilitation, or conventional hearing aids, which simply amplify the sound wave delivered to the ear, IHDs convert sound wave energy into kinetic energy, directly driving the ossicles of the middle ear. The sound energy is detected and received by a microphone. Then, through the use of either piezoelectric transduction or electromagnetic transduction, the sound energy from the environment is converted into mechanical energy that directly drives motion within the ossicles. Piezoelectric transduction occurs by converting the electrical charges produced by some forms of solid materials into energy producing a diaphragm or springboard effect.[41] These transducers tend to be precise, small, and accurate, typically requiring lower power. The disadvantage of this type of transducer is the requirement for fixation to the skull and ossicles, causing ossicular loading.[41] Electromagnetic transduction uses the motion of a magnet within an electrical field to drive the motion of the ossicles.[41] It does not require fixation to the skull, but it does generate a greater power requirement.[41] The IHDs are either completely implantable or semiimplantable (requiring an external component).

IHDs are indicated in individual with sensorineural, mixed, or conductive hearing loss.[42,43] One benefit of IHDs, particularly completely implantable devices, is the obviation of the need for a foreign body in the external auditory canal. Thus, patients with malformation of the external auditory canal, canal stenosis, irritation from earmold use, chronic otitis externa, eczema, or chronic disease of the outer ear may derive particular benefit from the completely implantable technologies.[43] These latter concerns are of particular interest within the geriatric population.

When compared with conventional hearing aids, there are a number of benefits associated with IHDs. They have been described to have better amplification capabilities with greater functional gain, improved sound quality, less distortion, more differentiated speech recognition, reduced feedback, improved perception in ambient conditions, and fewer complications from cerumen and ear canal occlusion.[41–43] For these reasons, implantable devices may be advantageous in the geriatric population with mild to severe hearing loss (up to approximately 80 dB).[42]

The Maxum implant (Ototronix, Saint Paul, MN), which consists of a rare earth magnet attached to the incudostapedial joint via a transcanal approach and an external deep in the ear device, has the advantage of avoiding high-frequency distortion, which can particularly be a problem in sloping presbycusic ears, and is often a complaint with conventional hearing aid users with this type of audiogram. A study evaluating 6 ears, average age of 67.5 years, implanted with the Maxum showed dramatic improvements in hearing and word recognition scores, with attendant improvements in quality of life, with patient-reported outcomes as satisfied (1/5) or very satisfied (4/5) compared with their best fit conventional hearing aids.[44]

The main disadvantage of IHDs is the obvious need for surgery. These devices may be implanted under general anesthesia or under local anesthesia with sedation, depending on the device selected. Elective exposure to general anesthesia is always a consideration in the geriatric population, particularly those with dementia. However, the duration and type of anesthesia is similar to that used for cochlear implantation, which has been well-established as safe in the geriatric population.[37–40] Additionally, the option of implanting certain devices under local anesthesia with sedation provides an exceptional alternative for patients with dementia where exposure to general anesthesia and the associated potential for progression of preexisting medical disease is of concern.

Additional disadvantages include ossicular disruption and device longevity. For certain devices, the ossicular chain must be irreversibly disrupted. This poses a significant potential disadvantage. Additionally, the device implanted and the power requirement may be inadequate as hearing severity increases. Given the limitations in acoustic output based on the required physical size of the device, there is a limitation in the severity of hearing loss that is amiable to implantable devices.[41] Patients may need to convert from an implanted acoustic device to a cochlear implant, depending on the progression of their hearing deficit. Additionally, these devices are typically not covered by most insurance providers. MRI compatibility is a concern for some devices, which is of greater importance in the geriatric population. **Table 1**

Table 1 Advantages and disadvantages of IHDs versus conventional hearing aids	
Advantages of IHDs	**Disadvantages of IHDs**
Superior amplification	Surgical requirement
Greater functional gain	Possible requirement of ossicular disruption
Improved sound quality	Uncertain device longevity
Decreased distortion	Limitations severity of hearing that may be implanted
Improved speech perception	With progression of hearing loss may require additional procedures (eg, CI)
Reduced feedback	MRI compatibility for certain devices
Improved perception in ambient conditions	
No cerumen complications	
Avoidance of canal occlusion/ occlusion effect	

Abbreviation: CI, cochlear implant; IHDs, implantable hearing devices.

provides a summary of the relative advantages and disadvantages of IHDs as compared with conventional hearing aids.

OSSEOINTEGRATED IMPLANTS

Another option for aural rehabilitation within the geriatric population with specific forms of hearing loss is the osseointegrated implant (OI). OIs require the surgical implantation of an implant within the calvarium that attaches or communicates with an external processor for the purpose of producing bone conduction auditory stimulation.

Geriatric patients who can derive benefit from OIs include those with conductive hearing loss, mixed hearing loss, and sensorineural hearing loss (single-sided deafness). Patients with conductive hearing loss with a cochlear reserve of 30 dB or better have the best performance with OIs, but patients do well with less cochlear reserve in mixed hearing loss. Within the geriatric population, conductive hearing loss may arise from a number of etiologies, including chronic ear disease, otosclerosis, or ossicular abnormalities (congenital or acquired). Mixed hearing loss may arise from any of these in combination with sensorineural hearing loss noted secondary to aging, head trauma, Meniere's disease, and other factors. There is a limitation in the available gain with OI, and patients should not be implanted for ipsilateral stimulation if there is a sensorineural component of 65 dB or more. It is important in counseling patients and selecting a device for aural rehabilitation to consider the current level of sensorineural hearing loss and likely anticipated progression in sensorineural hearing deficit. OI may also be used in the geriatric population with single-sided deafness of various etiologies (eg, sudden hearing loss, cerebellopontine angle tumors, birth defects/genetic disorders, trauma, Meniere disease, and adverse drug reactions) to direct sound to the better hearing ear. In a study of 21 patients with a mean age of 79 years (range, 65–88 years) after Baha implantation (Cochlear Americas, Centenial, CO) for single-sided deafness, auditory performance, and quality of life were evaluated.[45] All auditory parameters improved after implantation. When asked to relay their satisfaction level with a variety of features for their devices, patients reported primarily neutral or satisfied with their devices. Additionally, the Glasgow Benefit Inventory scores showed a 91% improved quality of life and the same 91% would recommend the procedure to others. **Table 2** presents the Glasgow Benefit Inventory results presented by Wazen and colleagues.[45]

The surgical procedure related to osseointegrated conduction devices may be performed with monitored sedation or general anesthesia. These procedures are usually performed in less than 1 hour. The main concern within the geriatric population is wound healing and potential cutaneous complications given the thin nature of skin in the geriatric population. Skin complication risk with percutaneous OIs is greater than with transcutaneous OIs, although it is low. For transcutaneous devices in the geriatric population, magnet intensity must be selected carefully to prevent skin complications secondary to excessive pressure.

There are a number of benefits from OI particularly in the geriatric population. Compared with conventional air conduction hearing aids, osseointegrated conduction implant devices obviate the need for occlusion of the ear canal.[46–49] This factor decreases the risk of chronic otorrhea and cerumen complication encountered with conventional air conduction hearing aids. Osseointegrated conduction implants done for mixed hearing loss, by directly stimulating the cochlea, also allow for less need for amplification as well as reduced occurrence of sound feedback.[46–49] Compared with traditional (nonimplanted) bone conduction hearing aids, they are reported to have increased comfort, better sound quality, and improved aesthetics.[50,51]

Table 2
Glasgow benefit inventory score in geriatric patients with OI for single-sided deafness

	All patients (n = 23)	Divino (n = 9)	Intenso (n = 14)
Total response score	18	20	17
General subscale	26	28	25
Social support	28	31	26
Physical health	12	13	12
Patients w/improved QOL	21 (91%)	9 (100%)	12 (86%)
Patients w/neutral or negative QOL	2 (9%)	0 (0%)	2 (7%)
Patients would recommend procedure	21 (91%)	8 (89%)	13 (93%)

Abbreviation: QOL, quality of life.
GBI scores range from −100 to +100, with −100 representing maximal negative benefit and +100 representing maximal positive benefit.
From Wazen JJ, VanEss MJ, Alameda J, et al. The Baha system in patients with single-sided deafness and contralateral hearing loss. Otolaryngol Head Neck Surg 2010;142:558; with permission.

SUMMARY

With the increasing aging population and projections of life expectancy ever increasing the elderly population with hearing loss will continue to increase. Hearing loss has a significant impact on quality of life, particularly in the elderly population, affecting an individual's psychological and cognitive well-being. Correction or augmentation of the hearing loss has been found to have a positive impaction of quality of life in the geriatric population. In addition to conventional hearing aids and cochlear implants, there are a number of safe and effective implantable options for aural rehabilitation within this population, depending on the type and severity of hearing loss. Patients and families should be counseled regarding their options to ensure informed medical decision making and optimization of quality of life.

REFERENCES

1. Frisina RD, Ding B, Zhu X, et al. Age-related hearing loss: prevention of threshold declines, cell loss and apoptosis in spiral ganglion neurons. Aging 2016;6: 2081–99.
2. Yueh B, Shapiro N, MacLean CH, et al. Screening and management of adult hearing loss in primary care: scientific review. JAMA 2003;289:1976–85.
3. Parham K, McKinnon BJ, Eibling D, et al. Challenges and opportunities in presbycusis. Otolaryngol Head Neck Surg 2011;144:491–5.
4. Mao Z, Zhao L, Pu L, et al. How well can centenarians hear? PLoS One 2013;8(6): e65565.
5. He W, Goodking D, Kowal P. An aging world: 2015. U.S. Census Bureau, International population reports, P25. Washington, DC: U.S. Government Publishing Office; 2016. p. 16–21.
6. Contrera KJ, Betz J, Li L, et al. Quality of life after intervention with a cochlear implant or hearing aid. Laryngoscope 2016;126:2110–5.
7. Li-Korotky HS. Age-related hearing loss: quality of care for quality of life. Gerontologist 2012;52:265–71.
8. Ciobra A, Bianchini C, Pelucci S, et al. The impact of hearing loss on the quality of life of elderly adults. Clin Interv Aging 2012;7:159–63.

9. Cacciatore F, Napoli C, Abete P, et al. Quality of life determinants and hearing function in an elderly population: Osservatorio Geriatrico Campano study group. Gerontology 1999;45:323–8.

10. Bernabei V, Morini V, Moretti F, et al. Vision and hearing impairments are associated with depressive-anxiety syndrome in Italian elderly. Aging Ment Health 2011; 15:467–74.

11. Uhlmann RF, Larson EB, Rees TS, et al. Relationship of hearing impairment to dementia and cognitive dysfunction in older adults. JAMA 1989;261:1916–9.

12. Kalayam B, Meyers MB, Kakuma T, et al. Age at onset of geriatric depression and sensorineural hearing deficits. Biol Psychiatry 1995;38:649–58.

13. Heine C, Browning CJ. Communication and psychosocial consequences of sensory loss in older adults: overview and rehabilitation directions. Disabil Rehabil 2002;24:736–73.

14. Dalton DS, Cruickshanks KJ, Klein BE, et al. The impact of hearing loss on quality of life in older adults. Gerontologist 2003;43:661–8.

15. Kramer SE, Kapteyn TS, Kuik DJ, et al. The association of hearing impairment and chronic diseases with psychosocial health status in older age. J Aging Health 2008;14:122–37.

16. Mohlman J. Cognitive self-consciousness – a predictor of increased anxiety following first-time diagnosis of age-related hearing loss. Aging Ment Health 2009;13:246–54.

17. Contrera KJ, Sung YK, Betz J, et al. Changes in loneliness after intervention with cochlear implants or hearing aids. Laryngoscope 2017;127:1885–9.

18. Choi JS, Betz J, Li L, et al. Association of using hearing aids or cochlear implants with changes in depressive symptoms in older adults. JAMA Otolaryngol Head Neck Surg 2016;142(7):652–7.

19. Uhlmann RF, Larson EB, Koepsell TD. Hearing impairment and cognitive decline in senile dementia of the Alzheimer's type. J Am Geriatr Soc 1986;34:207–10.

20. Weinstein BE, Amsel L. Hearing loss and senile dementia in the institutionalized elderly. Clin Gerontol 1986;4:3–15.

21. Herbst KG, Humphrey C. Hearing impairment and mental state in the elderly living at home. BMJ 1980;281:903–5.

22. LaForge RG, Spector WD, Sternberg J. The relationship of vision and hearing impairment to one-year mortality and functional decline. J Aging Health 1992;4: 126–48.

23. Ohta RJ, Carlin MF, Harmon BM. Auditory acuity and performance on the mental status questionnaire in the elderly. J Am Geriatr Soc 1981;29:476–8.

24. Peters CA, Potter JF, Scholer SG. Hearing impairment as a predictor of cognitive decline in dementia. J Am Geriatr Soc 1988;36:981–6.

25. Lindenberger U, Baltes PB. Sensory functioning and intelligence in old age: a strong connection. Psychol Aging 1994;9:339–55.

26. Gussekloo J, de Craen AJ, Oduber C, et al. Sensory impairment and cognitive functioning in oldest-old subjects: the Leiden 85+ Study. Am J Geriatr Psychiatry 2005;13:781–6.

27. Tay T, Wang JJ, Kifley A, et al. Sensory and cognitive association in older persons: findings from an older Australian population. Gerontology 2006;52:386–94.

28. Valentijn SA, van Boxtel MP, van Hooren SA, et al. Change in sensory functioning predicts change in cognitive functioning: results from a 6-year follow-up in the Maastricht Aging Study. J Am Geriatr Soc 2005;53:374–80.

29. Lin FR. Hearing loss and cognition among older adults in the United States. J Gerontol 2011;66A:1131–6.

30. Lin FR, Ferrucci L, Metter EJ, et al. Hearing loss and cognition in the Baltimore Longitudinal Study of Aging. Neuropsychology 2011;25:763–70.
31. Francis HW, Chee N, Yeagle J, et al. Impact of cochlear implants on the functional health status of older adults. Laryngoscope 2002;112:1482–8.
32. Olze H, Szczepek AJ, Haupt H, et al. Cochlear implantation has a positive influence on quality of life, tinnitus,and psychological comorbidity. Laryngoscope 2011;121:2220–7.
33. Mosnier I, Bebear JP, Marx M, et al. Improvement of cognitive function after cochlear implantation in elderly patients. JAMA Otolaryngol Head Neck Surg 2015;141:442–50.
34. Poissant SF, Beaudoin F, Huang J, et al. Impact of cochlear implantation on speech understanding, depression, and loneliness in the elderly. J Otolaryngol Head Neck Surg 2008;37:488–94.
35. Coelho DH, Yeh J, Kim JT, et al. Cochlear implantation is associated with minimal anesthetic risk in the elderly. Laryngoscope 2009;119:355–8.
36. Budenz CL, Cosetti MK, Coelho DH, et al. The effects of cochlear implantation on speech perception in older adults. J Am Geriatr Soc 2011;59:446–53.
37. Sanchez-Cuadro I, Lassaletta L, Perez-Mora RM, et al. Is there an age limit for cochlear implantation? Ann Otol Rhinol Laryngol 2013;122:222–8.
38. Lenarz M, Sonmez H, Joseph G, et al. Cochlear implant performance in geriatric patients. Laryngoscope 2012;122:1361–5.
39. Lin FR, Chien WW, Li L, et al. Cochlear implantation in older adults. Medicine (Baltimore) 2012;91:229–41.
40. Cosetti M, Lalwani A. Is cochlear implantation safe and effective in the elderly? Laryngoscope 2015;125(6):1279–81.
41. Blakely B. Hearing: when surgery is appropriate for age-related hearing loss. In: Geriatric care otolaryngology. American Academy of Otolaryngology-Head and Neck Surgery Foundation; 2006. p. 10–43. Available at: http://www.entnet.org/sites/default/files/Chapter-1_1.pdf. Accessed December 15, 2018.
42. Bittencourt AG, Burke PR, de Souza Jardim I, et al. Implantable and semi-implantable hearing aids: a review of history, indication, and surgery. Int Arch Otorhinolaryngol 2014;18:303–10.
43. Tisch M. Implantable hearing devices. GMS Curr Top Otorhinolaryngol Head Neck Surg 2017;16:Doc06.
44. Hunter JB, Carlson ML, Glasscock ME 3rd. The ototronix MAXUM middle ear implant for severe high-frequency sensorineural hearing loss: preliminary results. Laryngoscope 2016;126:2124–7.
45. Wazen JJ, VanEss MJ, Alameda J, et al. The Baha system in patients with single-sided deafness and contralateral hearing loss. Otolaryngol Head Neck Surg 2010;142:554–9.
46. Hol MK, Snik AF, Mylanus EA, et al. Long-term results of bone-anchored hearing aid recipients who had previously used air-conduction hearing aids. Arch Otolaryngol Head Neck Surg 2005;131:321–5.
47. McDermott AL, Dutt SN, Reid AP, et al. An intra-individual comparison of the previous conventional hearing aid with the bone-anchored hearing aid: the Nijmegen group questionnaire. J Laryngol Otol 2002;116:15–9.
48. DeWold MJ, Hedrick S, Creamers CW, et al. Better performance with bone anchored hearing aid that acoustic devices in patient with severe air-bone gap. Laryngoscope 2011;121:613–6.
49. Hol MK, Spath MA, Krabbe PF, et al. The bone-anchored hearing aid: quality of life assessment. Arch Otolaryngol Head Neck Surg 2004;130:394–9.

50. Hol MK, Kunst SJ, Snif AF, et al. Pilot study of the effectiveness of the conventional CROS, the transcranial CCROS and the BAHA transcranial CROS in adults with unilateral inner ear deafness. Eur Arch Otorhinolaryngol 2010;267:889–96.
51. Van der Pouw CTM, Snik AFM, Cremers CWRJ. The Baha HC200/300 in comparison with conventional bone conduction hearing aids. Clin Otolaryngol Allied Sci 1999;24:171–6.

Special Populations in Implantable Auditory Devices

Developmentally Challenged and Additional Disabilities

Daniel Jethanamest, MD[a],*, Baishakhi Choudhury, MD[b]

KEYWORDS

- Cochlear implants • Bone-anchored implants • Developmental delay
- Additional disabilities • Comorbidities • CHARGE

KEY POINTS

- Children with hearing loss and additional disabilities can benefit from cochlear implants and other implantable auditory devices.
- Auditory, speech, and language outcome measures show improvement over time when implantable auditory devices are used, although the rate of improvement and skill acquisition is typically slower than children without additional disabilities.
- For many children with hearing loss and additional disabilities, cochlear implants provide benefits to their quality of life; appropriate expectations should be considered for each individual child.
- Bone conduction devices provide benefit to populations with additional disabilities.

INTRODUCTION

Many children with significant hearing loss also have other disabilities. These disabilities may include developmental disabilities or cognitive impairment that can increase the complexity of the assessment for implantable auditory devices (IAD) as well as therapy and rehabilitation. Because children are receiving IAD including cochlear implants (CI) at earlier ages, many additional disabilities (ADs) may also not yet have been identified at the time of implantation, because some are not yet detectable during that early period.

Disclosure Statement: None.

[a] Division of Otology and Neurotology, Department of Otolaryngology–Head and Neck Surgery, NYU Langone Health, 550 First Avenue Suite 7Q, New York, NY 10016, USA; [b] Department of Otolaryngology Head and Neck Surgery, Loma Linda University Health, 11234 Anderson St. Rm 2586A, Loma Linda, CA 92354, USA

* Corresponding author.

E-mail address: Daniel.Jethanamest@nyumc.org

Although the prevalence of ADs can be difficult to assess, an estimated 15% to 40% of children with hearing impairment have an AD.[1–5] In one epidemiologic study, 27.4% of children with hearing loss were found to have at least one other disability, and in a study of the Metropolitan Atlanta Developmental Disabilities Surveillance Program, 30.4% of children had an AD.[6,7]

Developmental challenges and disabilities studied in children with IAD are varied in the types of disabilities, their relative effect on auditory performance, and in severity. Developmental delays (DD) may be identified when milestones are not met, including in the areas of motor skills, speech and language, cognition, social, and activities of daily living. Other nonauditory disabilities include autism spectrum disorder, cerebral palsy, neuropsychiatric disorders, visual disabilities, and learning disorders. In some cases, such as CHARGE syndrome, multiple disabilities and factors including anatomic inner ear dysplasias, nonauditory disabilities, and intellectual impairments may all contribute to more variable outcomes. Assessing children with complex needs and disabilities and counseling parents on the potential but variable benefits of IAD is challenging, and each case should be considered carefully and uniquely to assess the potential benefits attainable. Other than CI, there are very few to no papers looking at non-CI IADs in this population.

COCHLEAR IMPLANT OUTCOMES AND CONSIDERATIONS

Children with significant hearing loss and additional impairments may require more complex evaluations from a multidisciplinary team and careful counseling regarding expectations. Thorough access to rehabilitation and resources is also critical. Additional medical needs often delay evaluation and timing of CI compared with other children with profound hearing loss.[8] The assessment and diagnosis of DD and the trajectory of some disabilities may not present themselves clearly at young ages, so careful monitoring and assessment over time are important.

Auditory, Speech, and Language Benefits

Children with ADs as a heterogenous group have demonstrated benefits in outcomes, although with great variability. Lesinski and colleagues[3] reported on 108 children with ADs, 47 of whom were implanted. They proposed categorizing disabilities into those with direct influences on auditory perception, such as central processing disorders and autism, and those that were not directly related, and noted all the implanted children used their processors daily. Pyman and colleagues[9] compared 20 implanted children with motor and/or cognitive delay with another 55 implanted children with no delays, finding that the group with ADs overall progressed more slowly in speech perception levels. In 2000, Waltzman and colleagues[10] reported on 29 implanted children evaluated with a variety of closed and open-set speech perception measures, noting demonstrable benefits in auditory and linguistic skills and finding 59% used oral communication. Although this group showed a slower progression of auditory and linguistic skills, unmeasured improved social interactions and a general "connectedness" to the environment was observed. Birman and colleagues[2] reviewed Categories of Auditory Performance (CAP) in children with CI and ADs, compared with a group without other disabilities. CAP levels of 5 to 7 implied some verbal language, attained by 96% of those without ADs and 52% of the ADs group. The median CAP scores were significantly lower in those with DD than those without.

Studies have supported improvements in language skills with CI in this population, although the rate of improvement tends to be slower than peers. Meinzen-Derr and colleagues[11] evaluated receptive and expressive language outcomes using the Preschool

Language Scales. In a study of 20 children with CI and developmental disabilities, language measures did increase after CI; however, the rates of improvement were slow and as a group the median language quotients (normalization to chronologic age) did not improve. These investigators also compared this population with age/cognitive level–matched hearing controls, finding the group with ADs showed significantly lower mean receptive and expressive language measures.[12] Cruz and colleagues[1] reviewed the Childhood Development after Cochlear Implantation Study (CDaCI) cohort and identified 15% had an AD. Although all children showed continued language growth, those with ADs had a slower rate of improvement in both receptive and expressive oral language measures compared with those CI recipients without ADs.

Speech production outcomes have also been studied using the Speech intelligibility rating (SIR), a 5-point scale. Nikolopoulos and colleagues[13] compared long-term SIR outcomes for 67 children with ADs and with 108 without. At 5 years post-CI, 70% of the children with disabilities had connected intelligible speech, whereas 96% of those without disabilities achieved this level. Over time many of the children improve their intelligibility quite a bit, although the overall quality of speech was not as good—only 16% of the group with ADs achieved the 2 highest categorizations.

Reviewing 32 children with DD and CI, Edwards and colleagues[14] also used the SIR as well as E2L toy test and compared children with mild delays to those with significant DD. Those with mild delays had significantly better progress in developing speech in the years following CI. The finding that the severity of DD influences outcomes was also noted by Wakil and colleagues.[15] Updating long-term outcomes (7.3–19 years of CI use) for children with DD and CI, children with CI and severe DD were compared with those with mild to moderate DD. None of the children with severe DD developed open-set skills, whereas those with mild to moderate DD attained open-set speech perception scores ranging from 48% to 98%. Wiley and colleagues[5] noted the rate of progress on an Auditory Skills Checklist was similar for CI children with and without disabilities, but the progress significantly depended on the development level. Those with low developmental quotients had approximately half the rate of progress of typically developing CI children. Youm and colleagues[16] retrospectively compared 14 children with CI and intellectual disabilities (ID) with another 14 typical CI children. Among the ID group, 9 were identified as mild ID and 5 with moderate ID. Children in the mild group showed significant improvement in test parameters regarding auditory perception and language acquisition. However, children in the moderate group obtained limited benefit. Taken together, these studies suggest the severity of developmental or intellectual delays may be prognostic factors for auditory, speech perception, and intelligibility measures.

Cognitive, Functional, and Behavior Outcomes

Children with DD show a lower rate of intellectual development compared with CI recipients without DD. Oghalai and colleagues[8] assessed 204 children and studied 36 who completed all follow-up testing, including the Mullen Scales of Early Learning (MSEL), a measure used to estimate intelligence. They compared 12 children with DD to 24 without and found the DD group was on average implanted at an older age, possibly due to their complex medical needs. The CI group without disabilities improved in every domain of the MSEL and to a greater degree when compared with the DD group, which only improved in the fine motor domain. They also measured Vineland Adaptive Behavior Scales and noted that both groups showed appropriate developmental trajectories for age after CI, so the DD group did show a normal acquisition rate of adaptive behavior.

For children with complex needs and multiple disabilities, open-set speech perception and language development may not always be attainable or a primary goal. CI may provide other potential developmental benefits. Wiley and colleagues[17] used the Pediatric Evaluation of Disability Inventory (PEDI) to assess functional skills in 8 children with cognitive disabilities and CI. All of the children showed improvement in language skills; however, their rate of progress was not fast enough to keep up with their chronologic age. Similarly, the children made improvements in scale scores in all 3 PEDI domains after CI, although their median standard scores for the Self-care and Social Function domains decreased, indicating their rates of improvement were low and they would lose ground compared with chronologically matched peers over time. In an additional study of 14 children with CI compared with hearing controls with similar disabilities, the CI group showed similar PEDI scores for Self-care and Mobility but significantly lower scores for Social Function compared with the normal hearing children with similar disabilities.[18] This difference is likely due to language factors (nonverbal cognitive abilities and language level) because when these were controlled for, the difference was no longer significant. The CDaCI study evaluated internalizing and externalizing behavioral outcomes after CI. No increase in incidence of behavioral problems at baseline in children with ADs was found, but this group showed increases in externalizing behavior problems after CI compared with the group without ADs.[1]

Family-Reported Benefits and Quality of Life

Families and caretakers do perceive significant benefits of CI not easily conveyed by audiological or language tests. Wiley and colleagues[19] interviewed 15 families of children with multiple disabilities and CI, all of whom reported communication progress since the CI and would choose to have the CI if given the choice again. Parents reported that the majority (81%) was consistently using their CI devices, and 94% perceived their children developed awareness to environmental sounds. Berrettini and colleagues[20] studied 23 children with neuropsychiatric disorders and assessed speech perception in addition to adopting the questionnaire of Wiley and colleagues discussed earlier, in Italian. Preoperatively, 74% of the cohort was classified at the lowest categories (0–1) with none attaining category 6, whereas post-CI 53% achieved category 6 (open-set abilities). All the families reported their children had improved awareness of environmental sounds, 74% indicating improved speaking skills, and 96% reported improved interaction with peers.

Filipo and colleagues[4] also provided families or caretakers a questionnaire about the self-sufficiency of adults and children with CI and ADs, in addition to evaluating listening skills and social/family relationships. Listening skills and reported self-sufficiency improved while familial relationships remained stable. To better assess the benefits that CI may provide to this special population, Palmieri and colleagues[21] developed the Deafness and Additional Disabilities Questionnaire. This tool covers 5 areas: perceptual skills, preferred communication mode, communicative behaviors, attention/memory skills, and social interaction/control of behavior/self-government. They studied a group of 50 implanted children with ADs and found significant improvements across all 5 areas.

Speaker and colleagues[22] reported quality of life (QOL) benefits using the Glasgow Children's Benefit Inventory (GCBI) in a series of 16 children with profound and multiple learning disabilities. Very limited auditory improvements were seen, but positive QOL outcomes were noted—no respondents reported a negative impact of CI, 3 reported neither benefit nor harm, and the remainder were all positive.

CHARGE SYNDROME

Although many syndromes include hearing loss and ADs, CHARGE is one of the most common in the pediatric CI population. In addition to the classic findings of Coloboma,

Heart defects, choanal Atresia, Retardation, Genital anomalies, and Ear anomalies, additional anatomic findings may be seen in the brain stem, sella, clivus, and parotid.[23] Most relevant to CI, dysplasias of the semicircular canals and cochlea are common, often with an aberrant facial nerve and cochlear nerve deficiencies.[24] The presence of various elements of the phenotype varies considerably between patients, including a broad range of intelligence quotient and intellectual impairment, with approximately half having typical intellectual functioning.[25,26]

The studies performed on patients with CHARGE post-cochlear implantation have shown varied outcomes, as expected given the wide spectrum of abnormalities that can be found with the disorder. Some may also have a later age of implantation given their many complex medical conditions. In a study of 10 children with CHARGE syndrome implanted at 1 to 3.5 years of age, all showed some auditory benefit measured by audiometry and IT-MAIS.[27] Young and colleagues[28] reviewed 12 children with CHARGE and CI, categorizing auditory skills into 4 levels. Most achieved at least improved auditory detection, with 3 obtaining closed-set speech perception and 3 with open-set perception and noted cochlear nerve deficiency alone is not a contraindication to CI. These findings are consistent with other series that report improvements in at least auditory detection with a smaller, variable subset attaining improved speech perception.[29–31]

OTHER IMPLANTABLE AUDITORY DEVICES

Children with hearing loss and ADs may also be candidates for bone conduction implants (BCI) or other devices. Kunst and colleagues[32] have reported on their experience with 22 adult and pediatric patients with moderate ID. Benefit was reported on 2 separate parent- or caregiver-directed instruments, the GCBI, and the Listening Inventory for Education, which revealed results comparable to those of control BCI recipients without ID. Similarly, in 4 children with severe behavioral problems, the GCBI and an assessment of health status showed positive outcomes.[33] In a survey of providers for children with BCI and Down syndrome, a high rate of soft tissue complications was noted, but nevertheless a high perceived patient and care giver satisfaction was reported.[34] Pediatric auditory brainstem implants for patients who anatomically would not benefit from a CI show a varied range of auditory performance. A large proportion of these children have ADs distinct from hearing loss, which seems to be a negative prognostic factor for eventual auditory performance.[35]

SUMMARY

Children with hearing loss and additional disabilities should receive careful consideration for IADs and have demonstrated benefit across many measures. CI in this population has shown auditory and language benefits although typically their improvement is slower than peers without disabilities. In many cases, the potential benefits of auditory implants extend beyond auditory or language measures.

REFERENCES

1. Cruz I, Vicaria I, Wang N-Y, et al, CDaCI Investigative Team. Language and behavioral outcomes in children with developmental disabilities using cochlear implants. Otol Neurotol 2012;33(5):751–60.
2. Birman CS, Elliott EJ, Gibson WPR. Pediatric cochlear implants: additional disabilities prevalence, risk factors, and effect on language outcomes. Otol Neurotol 2012;33(8):1347–52.

3. Lesinski A, Hartrampf R, Dahm MC, et al. Cochlear implantation in a population of multihandicapped children. Ann Otol Rhinol Laryngol Suppl 1995;166:332–4.

4. Filipo, Bosco, Mancini, et al. Cochlear implants in special cases: deafness in the presence of disabilities and/or associated problems. Acta Otolaryngol 2004; 124(Suppl 552):74–80.

5. Wiley S, Meinzen-Derr J, Choo D. Auditory skills development among children with developmental delays and cochlear implants. Ann Otol Rhinol Laryngol 2008;117(10):711–8.

6. Fortnum HM, Marshall DH, Summerfield AQ. Epidemiology of the UK population of hearing-impaired children, including characteristics of those with and without cochlear implants–audiology, aetiology, comorbidity and affluence. Int J Audiol 2002;41(3):170–9.

7. Van Naarden K, Decouflé P, Caldwell K. Prevalence and characteristics of children with serious hearing impairment in metropolitan Atlanta, 1991-1993. Pediatrics 1999;103(3):570–5.

8. Oghalai JS, Caudle SE, Bentley B, et al. Cognitive outcomes and familial stress after cochlear implantation in deaf children with and without developmental delays. Otol Neurotol 2012;33(6):947–56.

9. Pyman B, Blamey P, Lacy P, et al. The development of speech perception in children using cochlear implants: effects of etiologic factors and delayed milestones. Am J Otol 2000;21(1):57–61.

10. Waltzman SB, Scalchunes V, Cohen NL. Performance of multiply handicapped children using cochlear implants. Am J Otol 2000;21(3):329–35.

11. Meinzen-Derr J, Wiley S, Grether S, et al. Language performance in children with cochlear implants and additional disabilities. Laryngoscope 2010;120(2):405–13.

12. Meinzen-Derr J, Wiley S, Grether S, et al. Children with cochlear implants and developmental disabilities: a language skills study with developmentally matched hearing peers. Res Dev Disabil 2011;32(2):757–67.

13. Nikolopoulos TP, Archbold SM, Wever CC, et al. Speech production in deaf implanted children with additional disabilities and comparison with age-equivalent implanted children without such disorders. Int J Pediatr Otorhinolaryngol 2008; 72(12):1823–8.

14. Edwards LC, Frost R, Witham F. Developmental delay and outcomes in paediatric cochlear implantation: implications for candidacy. Int J Pediatr Otorhinolaryngol 2006;70(9):1593–600.

15. Wakil N, Fitzpatrick EM, Olds J, et al. Long-term outcome after cochlear implantation in children with additional developmental disabilities. Int J Audiol 2014; 53(9):587–94.

16. Youm H-Y, Moon IJ, Kim EY, et al. The auditory and speech performance of children with intellectual disability after cochlear implantation. Acta Otolaryngol 2013; 133(1):59–69.

17. Wiley S, Meinzen-Derr J, Grether S, et al. Longitudinal functional performance among children with cochlear implants and disabilities: a prospective study using the pediatric evaluation of disability inventory. Int J Pediatr Otorhinolaryngol 2012; 76(5):693–7.

18. Meinzen-Derr J, Wiley S, Grether S, et al. Functional performance among children with cochlear implants and additional disabilities. Cochlear Implants Int 2013; 14(4):181–9.

19. Wiley S, Jahnke M, Meinzen-Derr J, et al. Perceived qualitative benefits of cochlear implants in children with multi-handicaps. Int J Pediatr Otorhinolaryngol 2005;69(6):791–8.

20. Berrettini S, Forli F, Genovese E, et al. Cochlear implantation in deaf children with associated disabilities: challenges and outcomes. Int J Audiol 2008;47(4): 199–208.
21. Palmieri M, Berrettini S, Forli F, et al. Evaluating benefits of cochlear implantation in deaf children with additional disabilities. Ear Hear 2012;33(6):721–30.
22. Speaker RB, Roberston J, Simoes-Franklin C, et al. Quality of life outcomes in cochlear implantation of children with profound and multiple learning disability. Cochlear Implants Int 2018;19(3):162–6.
23. Hoch MJ, Patel SH, Jethanamest D, et al. Head and neck MRI findings in CHARGE syndrome. AJNR Am J Neuroradiol 2017;38(12):2357–63.
24. Verloes A. Updated diagnostic criteria for CHARGE syndrome: a proposal. Am J Med Genet A 2005;133A(3):306–8.
25. Lasserre E, Vaivre-Douret L, Abadie V. Psychomotor and cognitive impairments of children with CHARGE syndrome: common and variable features. Child Neuropsychol 2013;19(5):449–65.
26. Raqbi F, Le Bihan C, Morisseau-Durand MP, et al. Early prognostic factors for intellectual outcome in CHARGE syndrome. Dev Med Child Neurol 2003;45(7): 483–8.
27. Lanson BG, Green JE, Roland JT, et al. Cochlear implantation in Children with CHARGE syndrome: therapeutic decisions and outcomes. Laryngoscope 2007; 117(7):1260–6.
28. Young NM, Tournis E, Sandy J, et al. Outcomes and time to emergence of auditory skills after cochlear implantation of children with charge syndrome. Otol Neurotol 2017;38(8):1085–91.
29. Vesseur A, Free R, Langereis M, et al. Suggestions for a guideline for cochlear implantation in CHARGE syndrome. Otol Neurotol 2016;37(9):1275–83.
30. Vincenti V, Di Lella F, Falcioni M, et al. Cochlear implantation in children with CHARGE syndrome: a report of eight cases. Eur Arch Otorhinolaryngol 2018; 275(8):1987–93.
31. Birman CS, Brew JA, Gibson WPR, et al. CHARGE syndrome and Cochlear implantation: difficulties and outcomes in the paediatric population. Int J Pediatr Otorhinolaryngol 2015;79(4):487–92.
32. Kunst SJW, Hol MK, Cremers CW, et al. Bone-anchored hearing aid in patients with moderate mental retardation: impact and benefit assessment. Otol Neurotol 2007;28(6):793–7.
33. Doshi J, McDermott A-L, Reid A, et al. The use of a bone-anchored hearing aid (Baha) in children with severe behavioural problems–the Birmingham Baha programme experience. Int J Pediatr Otorhinolaryngol 2010;74(6):608–10.
34. Sheehan PZ, Hans PS. UK and Ireland experience of bone anchored hearing aids (BAHA) in individuals with Down syndrome. Int J Pediatr Otorhinolaryngol 2006; 70(6):981–6.
35. Noij KS, Kozin ED, Sethi R, et al. Systematic review of nontumor pediatric auditory brainstem implant outcomes. Otolaryngol Head Neck Surg 2015;153(5):739–50.

Auditory Neuropathy
Bridging the Gap Between Hearing Aids and Cochlear Implants

Robert J. Yawn, MD, Ashley M. Nassiri, MD, MBA,
Alejandro Rivas, MD*

KEYWORDS

- Cochlear implant • Auditory neuropathy spectrum disorder • Hearing aid
- Hearing loss

KEY POINTS

- Auditory neuropathy spectrum disorder (ANSD) is a complex and heterogeneous disorder characterized by normal otoacoustic emissions and abnormal auditory brainstem response.
- A variety of treatment options exist for ANSD, including hearing amplification, cochlear implants (CI), or both.
- In patients with ANSD, younger age at time of cochlear implantation is associated with better audiologic outcomes.
- In patients with ANSD, cochlear nerve deficiency is associated with poor audiologic outcomes.

INTRODUCTION

Auditory neuropathy spectrum disorder (ANSD) is characterized by altered neural synchrony in response to auditory stimuli resulting in poor speech perception. The treatment of children with ANSD often requires a multidisciplinary approach with the involvement of teachers, family, otolaryngologists, audiologists, and speech and language pathologists. The variability in ANSD severity and response to treatment has created challenges in developing standardized treatments. For some

Disclosure Statement: A. Rivas: Consultant for Med-El, Advanced Bionics, Cochlear, Grace Medical, Stryker, and Cook Medical.
The Otology Group of Vanderbilt, Department of Otolaryngology–Head and Neck Surgery, Vanderbilt University Medical Center, 7209 Medical Center East, South Tower 1215 21st Avenue South, Nashville, TN 37232-8605, USA
* Corresponding author. Department of Otolaryngology–Head and Neck Surgery, The Bill Wilkerson Center for Otolaryngology and Communication Sciences, 7209 Medical Center East, South Tower, 1215 21st Avenue South, Nashville, TN 37232-8605.
E-mail address: alejandro.rivas@vanderbilt.edu

Otolaryngol Clin N Am 52 (2019) 349–355
https://doi.org/10.1016/j.otc.2018.11.016
0030-6665/19/© 2018 Elsevier Inc. All rights reserved.

oto.theclinics.com

patients, hearing amplification is adequate for appropriate auditory skill development, whereas others require cochlear implantation. This article describes the nuances in diagnosis and treatment of this patient population, with specific focus on factors that influence decision making when considering hearing amplification and cochlear implantation.

DIAGNOSIS

Children with ANSD classically present with uncharacteristically poor speech perception scores with respect to their auditory air-conduction pure tone threshold levels.[1] ANSD is a common disorder with an estimated prevalence of 5% to 15% of newborns with sensorineural hearing loss.[2–4] The cause of ANSD is believed to be related to neural dyssynchrony that leads to disruption of the processing of auditory signals at a variety of locations along the auditory pathway.[5] Locations implicated along the auditory pathway include the inner hair cells of the cochlea, the synapse between the inner hair cells and the cochlear nerve, and the ascending auditory nerve. The outer hair cells of the cochlea are not typically involved in ANSD. Patients with ANSD often present with normal otoacoustic emissions and absent or abnormal responses on auditory brainstem response (ABR) testing[1] with a robust cochlear microphonic with reversed stimulus polarity.[6] Furthermore, patients often have absent acoustic reflexes. Audiologic findings are summarized in **Table 1**.

Although the exact pathophysiology of auditory neuropathy is not completely understood, cochlear hypoxia has been proposed as a possible common factor among patients with ANSD.[7] Harrison[8] showed similar audiologic characteristics in animals with induced cochlear hypoxia and patients with ANSD. Besides hypoxia, the cause of ANSD may be multifactorial given its heterogeneity in severity and treatment outcomes. Ultimately, the pathogenesis seems to be related to a nonfatal insult to the inner hair cells that causes disruption of their connection to auditory neurons. Genetic mutations have also been investigated, with mutations in the OTOF and PJVK genes contributing to some sporadic cases of ANSD.[9]

Although ANSD can present in an otherwise healthy newborn, the clinician should be aware that it is often associated with other medical comorbidities including prematurity, hyperbilirubinemia, exchange transfusion, anoxia, developmental delay, mechanical ventilation, exposure to ototoxic drugs, low birth weight, infectious diseases, and various genetic disorders.[10] Identification and evaluation of comorbidities present in patients with ANSD is of paramount importance because these conditions can confound the diagnosis of ANSD and impact speech and language outcomes.

Table 1	
Diagnostic testing and characteristic clinical findings in ANSD	
Diagnostic Test	**Characteristic Findings in ANSD**
Auditory brainstem response	Absent or abnormal
Otoacoustic emissions	Normal
Cochlear microphonic	Robust with reversed polarity of stimulus
Acoustic reflexes	Absent
Pure tone thresholds	Normal to severe sensorineural hearing loss
Speech perception testing	Poor performance with respect to auditory threshold levels

TREATMENT
Hearing Aid Alone

Although the results of diagnostic testing are similar among ANSD patients, each case may vary in severity and response to treatment. This significant variability between patients creates challenges in creating a standardized treatment algorithm. After the diagnosis is confirmed with audiologic testing, most clinicians advocate for a trial with hearing aids (HAs) or an frequency modulation (FM) system, depending on the severity of hearing loss. The American Academy of Audiology recommends that children with ANSD should undergo a HA trial if auditory thresholds reveal that patients have inadequate speech perception at conversational levels.[11] Some studies have shown that ANSD patients that undergo HA trials have similar rates of speech and language development compared with similar age-matched patients with aidable sensorineural hearing loss.[12,13] Although some ANSD patients have significant benefit from HAs, performance does seem to be related to environmental noise. In quiet environments, patients with ANSD using HAs perform comparably with age-matched control subjects using HAs for sensorineural hearing loss. In noise, however, patients with ANSD perform significantly worse compared with their age-matched control subjects, which implicates neural dyssynchrony in creating difficulty in processing complex auditory signals.[11,13] Zeng and colleagues[14] hypothesize that this poor performance in noise is primarily related to altered timing-related perception and interaural time difference cues that lead to poor hearing and sound localization in complex environments.

Although HAs benefit some ANSD patients, there are some concerns with universal hearing amplification recommendations for ANSD patients. First, optimal fitting of HAs requires patient participation in behavioral testing to obtain behavioral thresholds. Given the high incidence of developmental delay in patients with ANSD, the inability to participate in behavioral testing can delay intervention. Second, it is possible that HAs may simply amplify an already distorted auditory signal without improving the underlying dyssynchrony, which can result in a lack of auditory skills development.[15,16] Third, there is a theoretic risk that sound amplification in ANSD patients, especially in the setting of absent acoustic reflexes and present cochlear microphonic, can place outer hair cells at increased risk of audiologic trauma and subsequent degradation.[16] Despite these concerns, if HAs are appropriately fitted and patient progress is monitored, many clinicians advocate for a trial of HA use before proceeding with more invasive treatment, such as cochlear implantation.

Cochlear Implantation

Cochlear implantation may be a treatment option in patients who have failed auditory skills development with traditional hearing amplification or in patients with both ANSD and unaidable profound sensorineural hearing loss. The exact means by which cochlear implantation improves speech and language performance in patients with ANSD is not completely understood. It is thought that cochlear implants (CIs) are able to restore synchronous firing in the neural pathway and increase the number of neural elements contributing to the ABR.[15] Animal models have also shown that increased neural synchrony is seen with electrical stimuli when compared with acoustic stimuli.[17] Another advantage attributed to electrical stimulation is increased access to speech cues, especially in patients with severe to profound hearing loss.[16,18]

Cochlear implantation for ANSD was first reported in a single case in 1999 by Rance and colleagues.[19] Although the patient in this case report had improved audiologic outcomes postoperatively, the outcomes were still poor compared with traditional implant candidates. Therefore, the perceived potential benefit from cochlear implantation in the ANSD population was initially believed to be low. A later study showed in a large cohort of 260 patients with ANSD that only 11% of patients with HAs alone showed subjective benefit versus 86% of patients with CIs[5]; however, this study was limited by the subjective nature of the outcomes measured. More recently, studies using objective criteria, such as speech perception testing, have shown that patients who demonstrate failure of auditory skills development with HAs alone do benefit from cochlear implantation.[20] A systematic review by Humphriss and colleagues[15] in 2013 analyzed 27 studies to evaluate the evidence for cochlear

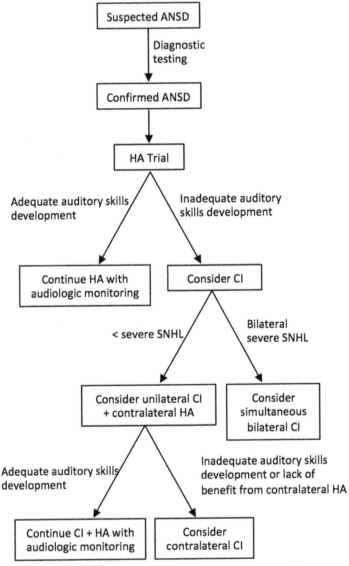

Fig. 1. A multidisciplinary approach to the evaluation of all patients with suspected auditory neuropathy spectrum disorder (ANSD) is preferred. CI, cochlear implant; HA, hearing aid; SNHL, sensorineural hearing loss.

implantation in ANSD and concluded that cochlear implantation leads to open-set speech perception in most patients. Furthermore, patients that fail HA trials achieve similar speech performance with cochlear implantation as those with ANSD that progress with HA use alone. Despite these findings, the authors of this review did conclude that the robustness of these conclusions is limited secondary to the heterogenous nature of the studies included.

Because of the inherent heterogeneity of disease severity and the resulting variability in performance after cochlear implantation, several studies have evaluated positive and negative prognostic factors for speech perception success after cochlear implantation surgery. Comorbid cochlear nerve deficiency has been identified as a significant negative factor in postoperative speech perception performance and overall benefit from cochlear implantation.[21] This has been identified in nearly one-quarter of patients with ANSD and, therefore, should be ruled out with imaging before proceeding with implantation.[22] Positive factors associated with improved performance are early age at diagnosis of ANSD and early age at implantation.[23] When compared with HAs alone, CIs are also associated with higher rates of cortical auditory evoked potentials, a measurement of cortical maturation.[24,25] Furthermore, children with implantation before 2 years of age are more likely to show age-appropriate cortical auditory evoked potentials responses within 6 months, suggesting a possible sensitive period for cortical auditory development.

Treatment Recommendations

Because of the considerable variability in disease severity and consequently the response to treatment in patients, developing a generalized treatment algorithm for patient with ANSD is challenging. The authors prefer a multidisciplinary approach to the evaluation of all patients with suspected ANSD (**Fig. 1**). Patients identified with hearing loss on newborn screening should be referred for audiologic and otolaryngologic work-up. If audiologic testing, particularly otoacoustic emissions and ABR testing, is suggestive of ANSD, patients should be evaluated for a HA trial. Where applicable, patients should be monitored with behavioral testing of auditory skills development to track progress. Additionally, input in the form of standardized surveys and evaluations should be gathered from family, teachers, and speech pathologists to assess for patient progress (**Table 2**). If patients fail to develop age-appropriate

Table 2
Speech perception testing

Questionnaires <2 y	Closed-Set >2 y	Open-Set Words >3–4 y	Open-Set Sentences >5 y
LittlEARS Auditory Questionnaire Parents' evaluation of Aural/Oral Performance of Children Scale Infant-Toddler Meaningful Auditory Integration Scale	Northwestern University-Children's Perception of Speech Early Speech Perception Test Pediatric Speech Intelligibility Test	Multisyllabic Lexical Neighborhood Test Consonant-Nucleus-Consonant words Northwestern University Auditory Test Phonetically Balanced Kindergarten words	Hearing in Noise Test for children AzBio sentence test adapted for children (BabyBio) Bromford-Kowal-Bench sentence lists

Suggested testing ages are based on patients with normal cognitive and developmental function.

language skills or continue to have poor audiologic performance, CI work-up should be considered. As a part of this evaluation, cochlear nerve deficiency or absence should be ruled out with MRI of the internal auditory canal. Patients with a present but deficient nerve can still undergo cochlear implantation, but parents should be appropriately counseled regarding the negative implications of this finding. Patients that do not progress with unilateral cochlear implantation should be considered for bilateral implantation with parental motivation and consent. The authors also consider sequential implantation in patients that have good performance with unilateral CI but limited benefit with contralateral HA, or in patients that stop using the contralateral HA after unilateral implantation. Patients that have undergone bilateral implantation at the authors' center have shown progression to open-set speech in some cases after failing to progress with unilateral cochlear implantation.

SUMMARY

Because of the heterogeneity of ANSD severity and high rates of comorbid developmental delay, patients with ANSD would benefit from individualized evaluation with respect to these factors. A tailored treatment plan may draw from a variety of options, including HAs, unilateral CI, bimodal hearing (CI plus HA), or bilateral cochlear implantation. A multidisciplinary approach with patient family involvement is beneficial in developing a treatment plan for each patient.

REFERENCES

1. Berlin CI, Morlet T, Hood LJ. Auditory neuropathy/dyssynchrony: its diagnosis and management. Pediatr Clin North Am 2003;50(2):331–40, vii-viii.
2. Kirkim G, Serbetcioglu B, Erdag TK, et al. The frequency of auditory neuropathy detected by universal newborn hearing screening program. Int J Pediatr Otorhinolaryngol 2008;72(10):1461–9.
3. Sanyelbhaa Talaat H, Kabel AH, Samy H, et al. Prevalence of auditory neuropathy (AN) among infants and young children with severe to profound hearing loss. Int J Pediatr Otorhinolaryngol 2009;73(7):937–9.
4. Mittal R, Ramesh AV, Panwar SS, et al. Auditory neuropathy spectrum disorder: its prevalence and audiological characteristics in an Indian tertiary care hospital. Int J Pediatr Otorhinolaryngol 2012;76(9):1351–4.
5. Berlin CI, Hood LJ, Morlet T, et al. Multi-site diagnosis and management of 260 patients with auditory neuropathy/dys-synchrony (auditory neuropathy spectrum disorder). Int J Audiol 2010;49(1):30–43.
6. Berlin CI, Bordelon J, St John P, et al. Reversing click polarity may uncover auditory neuropathy in infants. Ear Hear 1998;19(1):37–47.
7. Harrison RV, Gordon KA, Papsin BC, et al. Auditory neuropathy spectrum disorder (ANSD) and cochlear implantation. Int J Pediatr Otorhinolaryngol 2015; 79(12):1980–7.
8. Harrison RV. An animal model of auditory neuropathy. Ear Hear 1998;19(5): 355–61.
9. Wang J, Fan YY, Wang SJ, et al. Variants of OTOF and PJVK genes in Chinese patients with auditory neuropathy spectrum disorder. PLoS One 2011;6(9): e24000.
10. Bielecki I, Horbulewicz A, Wolan T. Prevalence and risk factors for auditory neuropathy spectrum disorder in a screened newborn population at risk for hearing loss. Int J Pediatr Otorhinolaryngol 2012;76(11):1668–70.

11. Walker E, McCreery R, Spratford M, et al. Children with auditory neuropathy spectrum disorder fitted with hearing aids applying the American Academy of Audiology pediatric amplification guideline: current practice and outcomes. J Am Acad Audiol 2016;27(3):204–18.

12. Ching TY, Day J, Dillon H, et al. Impact of the presence of auditory neuropathy spectrum disorder (ANSD) on outcomes of children at three years of age. Int J Audiol 2013;52(Suppl 2):S55–64.

13. Rance G, Barker EJ, Sarant JZ, et al. Receptive language and speech production in children with auditory neuropathy/dyssynchrony type hearing loss. Ear Hear 2007;28(5):694–702.

14. Zeng FG, Kong YY, Michalewski HJ, et al. Perceptual consequences of disrupted auditory nerve activity. J Neurophysiol 2005;93(6):3050–63.

15. Humphriss R, Hall A, Maddocks J, et al. Does cochlear implantation improve speech recognition in children with auditory neuropathy spectrum disorder? A systematic review. Int J Audiol 2013;52(7):442–54.

16. Rance G. Auditory neuropathy/dys-synchrony and its perceptual consequences. Trends Amplif 2005;9(1):1–43.

17. Dynes SB, Delgutte B. Phase-locking of auditory-nerve discharges to sinusoidal electric stimulation of the cochlea. Hear Res 1992;58(1):79–90.

18. Buss E, Labadie RF, Brown CJ, et al. Outcome of cochlear implantation in pediatric auditory neuropathy. Otol Neurotol 2002;23(3):328–32.

19. Rance G, Beer DE, Cone-Wesson B, et al. Clinical findings for a group of infants and young children with auditory neuropathy. Ear Hear 1999;20(3):238–52.

20. Pelosi S, Wanna G, Hayes C, et al. Cochlear implantation versus hearing amplification in patients with auditory neuropathy spectrum disorder. Otolaryngol Head Neck Surg 2013;148(5):815–21.

21. Freeman SR, Stivaros SM, Ramsden RT, et al. The management of cochlear nerve deficiency. Cochlear Implants Int 2013;14(Suppl 4):S27–31.

22. Roche JP, Huang BY, Castillo M, et al. Imaging characteristics of children with auditory neuropathy spectrum disorder. Otol Neurotol 2010;31(5):780–8.

23. Dean C, Felder G, Kim AH. Analysis of speech perception outcomes among patients receiving cochlear implants with auditory neuropathy spectrum disorder. Otol Neurotol 2013;34(9):1610–4.

24. Rance G, Cone-Wesson B, Wunderlich J, et al. Speech perception and cortical event related potentials in children with auditory neuropathy. Ear Hear 2002;23(3):239–53.

25. Sharma A, Cardon G, Henion K, et al. Cortical maturation and behavioral outcomes in children with auditory neuropathy spectrum disorder. Int J Audiol 2011;50(2):98–106.

Implantable Auditory Devices

Financial Considerations and Office-Based Implantation

Jack Wazen, MD[a,b,*], Joshua Smith, DO[c],
Julie Daugherty, PhD, NP-C[d]

KEYWORDS

- BAHA • Implantable hearing devices • Middle ear implant • Cost-effectiveness

KEY POINTS

- Medicare and the third-party payers must declassify implantable hearing devices as hearing aids and instead place them under prosthetic devices such as cochlear implants, cataracts, hips, and knees.
- Office-based placement of implantable auditory devices requires careful patient selection and preoperative planning to obtain optimal outcomes.
- A range of device options is suitable for office placement, including both osseointegrated implants and partially implantable hearing aids.

FINANCIAL CONSIDERATIONS

The explosion in technological advances we are witnessing has revolutionized our day-to-day lives. Our phones and watches are minicomputers; we can listen to our favorite tunes anywhere on our smart devices, no more records or CDs necessary. Our cars are computerized and can take us anywhere by just typing in an address. This accelerated progress in technology has also transformed health care delivery. Information technology has enhanced the operational efficiency of the medical team, improving patient safety and the standards of care. Moreover, the Internet has allowed rapid dissemination of the latest clinical data regarding disease symptomology and treatment outcomes to both the consumer and the clinician. In some specialty areas

Disclosure Statement: None of the authors have any disclosures to report.
[a] Department of Surgery, Division of Otolaryngology Head and Neck Surgery, Sarasota Memorial Hospital, 1901 Floyd street, Sarasota, Florida 34239, USA; [b] Silverstein Institute, 1901 Floyd Street, Sarasota, FL 34239, USA; [c] Otology, Silverstein Institute, 1901 Floyd Street, Sarasota, FL 34239, USA; [d] Research for the Ear Research Foundation, Silverstein Institute, 1901 Floyd Street, Sarasota, FL 34239, USA
* Corresponding author. Silverstein Institute, 1901 Floyd Street, Sarasota, FL 34239.
E-mail address: jwazen@earsinus.com

of health care, the widespread use of technology and consumer demand has lowered costs of some services, improving the patient's access to vital medical care. Unfortunately, such benefits have not translated into the hearing rehabilitation field. Although there have been significant technological developments in the hearing device industry that offer great benefit for patients with hearing loss, factors including stigma and cost continue to be barriers.

It is estimated that 67% to 86% of adults (50 years and older) who may benefit from hearing aids do not use them, and many hearing assistive technologies as well as auditory rehabilitation services are not fully used. The concept of stigma associated with hearing loss (and hearing devices) has been described extensively in previously published literature. Qualitative research suggests an individual forms a "perceived stigma," from societal biases and preconceptions of hearing devices. This stigma affects their initial acceptance of hearing loss and decision for seeking testing and treatment. In addition, alteration in self-perception, ageism, and vanity also contribute to the development of stigma.[1]

In 2016, The National Academies of Sciences, Engineering, and Medicine convened an expert committee to study the accessibility and affordability of hearing health care for adults in the United States.

The committee-identified gaps or deficiencies recommended key institutional, technological, and regulatory changes that would enable consumers to find and fully use the appropriate, affordable, and high-quality services, technologies, and supports they need. They acknowledged hearing loss as an important medical issue for individuals (and to some extent their families and friends) as well as the recognition that it is a significant public health concern that has to be addressed by actions at multiple levels.[2]

The committee concluded that improving the accessibility and affordability of hearing health care will require a collaborative organizational effort in the public and private sectors and across professions. Since the publication of this report, the Food and Drug Administration (FDA) has cleared the way for the "over-the-counter hearing aids" to be added to the personal sound amplification products (PSAP) for mild hearing losses without the need for a medical clearance.

When it comes to implantable hearing devices, financial considerations play an even bigger role due to the higher expenses added such as surgical, anesthesia, and hospital fees. We are grateful that cochlear implants have been covered by the third party payers for a while now. We are also grateful that after many years of being FDA approved, osseointegrated auditory implants are now covered by Medicare and most insurance carriers. Medicare, however, attempted withdrawing coverage for the osseointegrated implants a few years ago but reconsidered and maintained coverage after being deluged by objection letters from professional societies, and consumer organizations and networks, a proof that there is strength in multidisciplinary collaboration.

Reducing health care costs is everyone's duty. One way to lower surgical costs is to provide the services in the doctor's offices instead of in hospitals or ambulatory surgery centers, thus eliminating hospital and facility fees as well as anesthesia costs.[3] Osseointegrated auditory systems can be easily performed in the office under local anesthesia. The main stumbling block, however, is the insurance industry that would benefit most from the cost savings! Purchasing the implants and processors needs to be made possible and unbundled through the doctor's offices.

The other major deterrent for patients receiving implantable auditory devices, or even hearing aids, is the lack of insurance coverage. Medicare continues to deny coverage for all hearing rehabilitation devices except for cochlear implants and osseointegrated implants based on their definition as hearing aids. Multiple attempts to reclassify implantable hearing devices as prosthetics to be used when hearing aids have failed have not been successful. Although it is well within Medicare's purview to do so, they have so far resisted the change transferring the responsibility to Congress, a long and winding road.

So, in summary, in order for more subjects to accept hearing rehabilitation, the following need to happen:

- The prices must come down.
- Short procedures that are feasible under local anesthesia should be done in the doctor's office.
- Medicare and the third-party payers must declassify implantable hearing devices as hearing aids and place them under prosthetic devices such as cochlear implants, cataracts, hips, and knees.

OFFICE-BASED IMPLANTATION

The evolution of implantable auditory devices and refinement of surgical technique have allowed surgeons to offer implantation in the office as a safe, convenient, and potentially cost-saving option.[3] Although a variety of implantable devices are commercially available,[4] there are a limited number that lend themselves readily to office-based surgical approaches. Procedures that are more invasive involve elevation of large skin flaps or extensive subcutaneous dissection are more suited for the controlled environment of an operating theatre. Therefore, this discussion is limited to those devices that are most easily and readily implanted in the office setting. **Table 1** lists the FDA-approved implants that most readily lend themselves to office placement. These include the MAXUM system (Ototronix LLC, Houston, Texas, USA), the Cochlear Baha (Cochlear Americas, Denver, Colorado, USA), and Oticon/Ponto (Oticon Medical AB, Askim, Sweden).

Considerations for Office-Based Implantation

Important factors common to all office-based surgical procedures:

1. Patient selection: proper patient selection is one of the primary determinants of success in office-based surgery. Multiple factors must each be carefully considered, including patient anxiety, expectations, anatomic considerations,[5] and prior ear surgery or radiation. Comorbid conditions such as poorly controlled diabetes, bleeding disorders (or use of blood thinners), and immunocompromised state must be carefully considered.
2. Office Staff: proper training of office staff is crucial. They must be familiar with sterile technique, the procedure itself, and the instrumentation to be used.
3. Anesthesia: the combination of oral and local anesthesia will be more than adequate in most cases. Patients may be premedicated with an anxiolytic such

Table 1	
Summary of implantable auditory devices available for office implantation	
Osseointegrated Implant	**Partially/Totally Implantable Hearing Aids**
Baha Connect, Attract (Cochlear)	MAXUM (Ototronix)
Minimally Invasive Ponto Surgery (Oticon)	

as diazepam, lorazepam, or triazolam. Preoperative discussion of patient expectations is crucial in lessening patient anxiety.

4. Equipment: it is prudent to equip an office procedure room with a standard "crash cart" in the event of an unexpected complication requiring defibrillation or advanced airway placement. Particularly when using staff who initially may be inexperienced, the risk having to terminate a procedure due to dropping or contaminating instruments can be mitigated by making backup equipment readily available.

Osseointegrated Implants

There has been a significant evolution of surgical technique in the placement of osseointegrated implants throughout the past several decades.[6] Historically, the surgical procedure consisted of extended soft tissue dissection with an increased incidence of postoperative wound complications and less cosmetically favorable outcomes. These stages included the following: (1) implantation of the titanium implant with abutment into the temporal bone (conventionally on the mastoid process); (2) soft tissue reduction around the implant site using various techniques including full-thickness skin grafting and pedicled split-thickness skin flaps; and (3) eExteriorizing the implant with the abutment in a single stage or as a 2-stage procedure.[7] As noted earlier, Cochlear (Cochlear Americas, Denver, Colorado, USA) and Oticon (Oticon Medical AB, Askim, Sweden) both produce implants that are conducive to office-based surgery. The Cochlear Connect, Cochlear Attract, and the Oticon Minimally Invasive Ponto Surgery (MIPS) are discussed. Patients who require soft tissue reduction or have a scalp thickness of more than 1 cm should not have their osseointegrated implant placed in the office. Procedure time and risk of bleeding increase with soft tissue dissection. Placement of the Cochlear Attract requires the elevation of a small skin flap. Some practitioners may choose not to offer this procedure in the office because of the increased soft tissue dissection compared with the Connect device. When planning for placement of the Oticon MIPS or Cochlear Connect, a range of abutment sizes should be made available before starting the procedure, even if the patient's skin thickness has been previously measured. Many practitioners routinely use transcutaneous methylene blue to score and stain the periosteum at the selected implant site. Placement of the implant along the temporal line where the cortical bone is thickest facilitates consistent placement, avoidance of mastoid air cells, and optimal bone stock for single-stage surgery. Surgical guides with manufacturer recommendations for implant placement technique are readily available.

Partially Implantable Hearing Aids

Many of the drawbacks of conventional hearing aids are a result of the limitations of sound transmission through the external auditory canal. Chief among these is inadequate gain in the higher frequencies for patients with severe downsloping sensorineural hearing loss.[8] Other limitations include the social stigma of an externally visible hearing aid, frequent battery replacement, frequent cleaning and maintenance, cerumen impaction, and inability to submerge the head with the hearing aids in place.[9] These and other concerns led to the development of implantable hearing devices. The Vibrant Soundbridge (Med-El Corporation, Innsbruck, Austria) was the first partially implantable hearing aid to receive FDA approval and was released in 2003, targeting patients with moderate to severe sensorineural hearing loss.[4] Multiple device options are available today. The Esteem (Envoy Medical Corporation, Minnesota, USA) and Vibrant Soundbridge (Med-El Corporation, Innsbruck, Austria) require a mastoidectomy with facial recess dissection for implant placement. The MAXUM (Ototronix

LLC Houston, Texas, USA), which was released in 2009, is a partially implantable auditory device and consists of both an internal implantable device and an external processor. The external processor fits within the external auditory canal and is customized based on preoperative molds of the patient's canal. Motivated patients with exostoses, canal stenosis, or a tortuous canal may require canaloplasty in order to successfully proceed with MAXUM (Ototronix LLC Houston, Texas, USA) fitting and placement.[10] The implant is magnetic and requires the use of nonmagnetic instruments to position and manipulate the magnet onto the ossicular chain. These must be kept separate from instruments that can become magnetized to avoid potential avulsion injury of the ossicular chain in the event of magnet mobilization with a conventional instrument. A small Skeeter type drill should also be made available if necessary for widening the posterosuperior ear canal for better visualization and access to the incudostapedial joint.

SUMMARY

Hearing rehabilitation has been recognized as a crucial tool to maintain communicative and social skills. The availability of hearing aids and auditory implants ought not be limited to the wealthy and to those who can afford them. Multidisciplinary efforts in reducing costs are necessary and include reduction of the item costs, insurance coverage, and the ability to perform certain procedures in an office setting, eliminating hospital and facilities fees and anesthesia bills.

REFERENCES

1. Wallhagen MI. The stigma of hearing loss. Gerontologist 2010;50(1):66–75.
2. Strawbridge WJ, Wallhagen MI, Shema SJ, et al. Negative consequences of hearing impairment in old age: a longitudinal analysis. Gerontologist 2000; 40(3):320–6.
3. Catalano PJ, Choi E, Cohen N. Office versus operating room insertion of the bone-anchored hearing aid: a comparative analysis. Otol Neurotol 2005;26(6): 1182–5.
4. Bittencourt AG, Burke PR, Jardim Ide S, et al. Implantable and semi-implantable hearing AIDS: a review of history, indications, and surgery. Int Arch Otorhinolaryngol 2014;18(3):303–10.
5. Berenholz LP, Burkey JM, Lippy WH. High body mass index as a risk factor for skin overgrowth with the bone-anchored hearing aid. Otol Neurotol 2010;31(3): 430–2.
6. van de Berg R, Stokroos RJ, Hof JR, et al. Bone-anchored hearing aid: a comparison of surgical techniques. Otol Neurotol 2010;31(1):129–35.
7. Verheij E, Bezdjian A, Grolman W, et al. A systematic review on complications of tissue preservation surgical techniques in percutaneous bone conduction hearing devices. Otol Neurotol 2016;37(7):829–37.
8. Hunter JB, Carlson ML, Glasscock ME 3rd. The ototronix MAXUM middle ear implant for severe high-frequency sensorineural hearing loss: preliminary results. Laryngoscope 2016;126(9):2124–7.
9. Memari F, Asghari A, Daneshi A, et al. Safety and patient selection of totally implantable hearing aid surgery: Envoy system, Esteem. Eur Arch Otorhinolaryngol 2011;268(10):1421–5.
10. Pelosi S, Carlson ML, Glasscock ME 3rd. Implantable hearing devices: the Ototronix MAXUM system. Otolaryngol Clin North Am 2014;47(6):953–65.

Future of Implantable Auditory Devices

Robert M. Rhodes, MD, Betty S. Tsai Do, MD*

KEYWORDS

- Totally implantable • Robotic • Cochlear implants
- Microelectromechanical systems • Future

KEY POINTS

- Engineering and medical collaboration are at the forefront of auditory device advancement.
- Totally implantable auditory devices are being affected by improvements in microelectronic system design.
- Alternative energy sources for cochlear implant array stimulation of the spiral ganglion may lead to optimal hearing outcomes.
- Drug-eluting and drug-delivering cochlear implant arrays may improve short-term and long-term hearing outcomes.
- Robotic-assisted and robotically performed otologic surgery has the potential to improve outcomes and decrease morbidity.

INTRODUCTION

Technological innovations are continuing to enhance human existence and provide exciting ways in which people interact with their surroundings. In 2006, Jackler[1] described the stigma of hearing aid devices, attributable to their association with older age and even possible intellectual disability. Since then, society has continued to see certain hearing devices become more socially accepted and part of everyday life; for instance, the movie screen example of the successful, middle-aged businessman wearing an earpiece for communication. The continued, rapid technological advancements of cellular phones residing in consumers' pockets are now dually serving as powerful central processing units with endless capabilities. This advance creates limitless possibilities for the development of earpiece-centered interactive devices. As

Disclosure: Advanced Bionics (B.S. Tsai Do), principal investigator of clinical trial for multicenter electroacoustic stimulation study; R.M. Rhodes has nothing to disclose.
The Department of Otolaryngology Head and Neck Surgery, The University of Oklahoma Health Sciences Center, 800 Stanton L Young Boulevard, Suite 1400, Oklahoma City, OK 73104, USA
* Corresponding author.
E-mail address: betty.tsai@gmail.com

the stigma of hearing amplification continues to fade, it is hoped that the self-consciousness will concurrently decline and the percentage of patients using hearing amplification devices will increase.

Multidisciplinary research among medical and engineering fields will continue to be critical in the development of new technology to increase the number of hearing amplification candidates using hearing devices. The foreseeable future is likely to include smaller, more efficient, interactive hearing devices, some of which will be fully implantable, depending on patients' wishes. In addition, alternative energy sources continue to be investigated to improve system efficiency and sound clarity. The ultimate goal is improved quality of life and societal interactions to the appropriate patient candidates while also contributing to a sustainable health care economy. Secondarily, harnessing the impact of new technological developments may lead to avenues for a more convenient and entertaining human experience through the development of recreational hearing devices.

IMPLANTABLE SENSORS

The limitations of hearing aids are discussed in Sara Lerner's article, "Limitations of Conventional Hearing Aids – Examining Common Complaints and Issues that Can and Cannot be Remedied," in this issue. To overcome some of the limitations, alternative ways of driving the tympanic membrane and ossicular chain were explored, resulting in the development of middle ear implants and other active osseointegrated devices. These devices take advantage of using implantable sensors of different varieties that broaden the dynamic and frequency range compared with conventional aids. These implantable sensors have allowed the prototypes and development of partially and totally implantable hearing aids, which includes totally implantable middle ear implants and eventually totally implantable cochlear implants. As human hearing includes a range from 20 Hz to 20 kHz, with speech primarily constrained from 250 to 8 kHz and environmental sounds with a lower frequency limit of 100 Hz; an ideal range for the sensor would be from 100 Hz to 8 kHz. However, biocompatibility, size and mass limitations, and power consumption must be taken into account in the design of these sensors.

Although not an implant in the truest form, the simplest use of implantable sensors is that seen in the Earlens device, which uses a lens overlying the tympanic membrane to convert light energy into an electrical current (**Fig. 1**A), driving the umbo from the

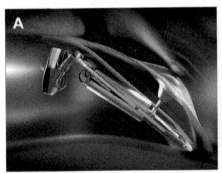 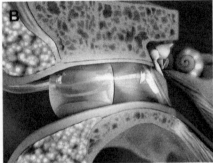

Fig. 1. The Earlens device. (*A*) A custom-fitted lens is placed and adheres to the tympanic membrane using surface tension. (*B*) Sound enters the microphone and is converted to nonvisible light using a photon processor that delivers this energy to the lens. (*Courtesy of* Earlens, Menlo Park, CA; with permission.)

lateral side of the tympanic membrane. Sound is captured from a behind-the-ear processor and transformed to nonvisible light energy within the external auditory canal. This light energy is subsequently directed at a detector on the lens, which converts the light into a mechanical driving force directly applied to the tympanic membrane, as shown in **Fig. 1**B.[2] The described major advantage is the device's ability to provide amplification, up to 68 dB, over a broad frequency range of 125 Hz to 10,000 Hz, which is a limitation of the current air-conduction hearing aids.[3]

More recently, MEMS (microelectromechanical systems) technology has been used to develop subcutaneous sensors using similar principles to conventional hearing aids but with a significantly smaller footprint.[4] Because of its small size, this technology has been used as prototypes for totally implantable middle ear implants and, more recently, as a sensor for intracochlear pressure.[5,6] Similarly, piezoelectric sensors, made from materials that deform when small differences in electrical voltage are applied, have been integrated into the development of totally implantable hearing aids, such as the Esteem. A piezoelectric microphone that can be inserted into the round window to detect pressure changes within the cochlea from sound stimuli has been developed as a precursor to a totally implantable cochlear implant.[7] By merging the two technologies into a piezoelectric MEMS accelerometer, smaller sensors with low power consumption are possible with bandwidths up to 20 kHz: the upper range of human hearing.[4] Examples of such sensors have already been developed in artificial basilar membranes that can be implanted into the cochlea and use vibrations to generate current to stimulate spiral ganglion cells.[8,9] This development could pave the way for totally implantable cochlear implants.

DIRECT ACOUSTIC COCHLEAR IMPLANT

Although middle ear implants and bone conduction implants continue to play important roles for patients with conductive and mixed hearing losses, they lack the ability to provide adequate stimulation for patients with a significant amount of sensorineural hearing loss. Active middle ear implants such as the Bonebridge are described in C. Y. Joseph Chang's article, "Ossicle Coupling Active Implantable Auditory Devices: Magnetic Driven System" and Michael D. Seidman and colleagues' article, "Totally Implantable Active Middle Ear Implants," in this issue. However, a direct acoustic cochlear implant was first presented in 2008 and takes it one step further.[10] Intended for patients with advanced otosclerosis, the device consists of a stapes piston attached to an artificial incus driven by an electromagnetic transducer (also referred to as the direct acoustic cochlear stimulator [DACS]) to directly stimulate the perilymph with an external behind-the-ear audio processor. This initial trial of 4 patients showed significant improvement in monosyllabic word recognition scores (by 45–100 percentage points) for patients whose initial hearing thresholds were in the 78 to 101 dB pure-tone average range. Although initially 2 different versions of this investigational device were created, 1 using the Cochlear Freedom processor (commonly referred to as the Codacs) and another using a processor provided by Phonak Acoustic Implants (referred to as the direct acoustic cochlear stimulation partial implant), only the Codacs has continued to undergo clinical trials.[11,12] **Fig. 2** shows the current Codacs system undergoing clinical trials in Europe.[13]

The first Codacs trial was a multicenter trial of 15 patients with advanced otosclerosis with a severe to profound mixed hearing loss and who had previously failed a stapedectomy.[12] Surgery consisted of a transmastoid and transcanal or posterior tympanotomy approach in order to adequately access the stapes footplate. Similar

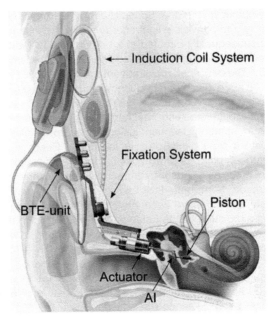

Fig. 2. The Codacs system. Sound input enters through a behind-the-ear (BTE) processor to communicate with the internal receiver through an induction coil system similar to that of a cochlear implant. A piston through the stapes footplate is connected to the artificial incus (AI), which is driven by an actuator controlled by the Cochlear Nucleus Freedom platform. The device is secured to the mastoid by a fixation system. (*From* Grossohmichen M, Salcher R, Kreipe HH, et al. The Codacs direct acoustic cochlear implant actuator: exploring alternative stimulation sites and their stimulation efficiency. PLoS One 2015;10(3):e0119601; with permission; and *Courtesy of* Cochlear Limited, Sydney, Australia.)

to middle ear implants, surgical time decreased with surgeon experience, with the average surgery averaging nearly 5 hours for 15 patients, but this had decreased to 2.5 hours by the eighth patient.[12]

Surgery did not change the air-conduction or bone-conduction thresholds, with a mean unaided threshold of 86 dB. With the Codacs device, the mean threshold was 38 dB. For patients who used a hearing aid, the mean unaided threshold was 83 dB and 37 dB with the Codacs device compared with 52 dB with a hearing aid. The greatest gain was seen at 1500 Hz. In addition, word recognition scores improved by 36% at 50 dB of sound pressure level (SPL), 77.3% 65 dB SPL, and 80.2% at 80 dB SPL compared with the unaided preoperative condition.[12]

Since the initial multicenter trial, there have been cadaveric studies exploring different sites of stimulation as well as studies in patients for other indications. Although the Codacs device stimulates the inner ear through a stapes piston (**Fig. 2**), alternative stimulation sites, such as the round window, stapes head with a bell prosthesis, and even an aerial prosthesis over the stapes footplate, have been found to be adequate potential sites based on temporal bone studies (**Fig. 3**).[13] According to temporal bone studies, stimulation at the round window was similar in output to the piston, whereas stimulation with the stapes head with the bell prosthesis and the footplate with the aerial prosthesis was more efficient. However, the investigators noted that a redesign of the Codacs system would be required in order for these new systems to work because of space constraints within the middle ear.

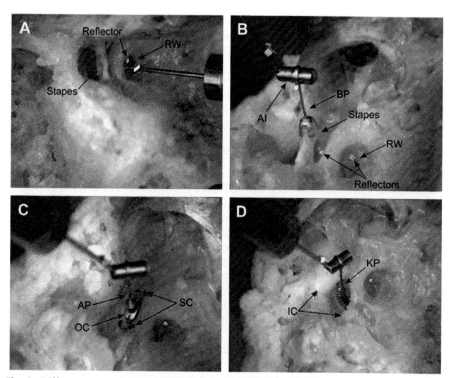

Fig. 3. Different potential methods of stimulating the inner ear through temporal bone studies. Reflectors are placed within the temporal bone to measure movement within the inner ear caused by various methods of stimulation. (*A*) Stimulation through the round window (RW). (*B*) A bell prosthesis (BP) is used to attach to the stapes head in order to stimulate the inner ear. (*C*) An aerial prosthesis (AP) is connected to an omega connector (OC) as a ball joint and placed on the stapes footplate. (*D*) A piston through a stapedotomy after the footplate has been fixed by ionomer cement (IC) to simulate otosclerosis. This configuration is used in the Codacs device when used in advanced otosclerosis. KP, K-Piston prosthesis (0.4 × 5.0 mm, Heinz Kurz GmbH Medizintechnik, Germany); SC, stapes crura. (*From* Grossohmichen M, Salcher R, Kreipe HH, et al. The Codacs direct acoustic cochlear implant actuator: exploring alternative stimulation sites and their stimulation efficiency. PLoS One 2015;10(3):e0119601; with permission; and *Courtesy of* Cochlear Limited, Sydney, Australia.)

Therefore, there is a possibility that after redesign the coupling efficiency is not as good as that of the current Codacs system.

Initial indications for the Codacs system were for patients with a severe to profound mixed hearing loss in the setting of otosclerosis. Since then, implantation for alternative disorders has been shown to be successful in other patients. Schwab and colleagues[14] placed the Codacs system in 4 patients whose mastoids were obliterated with fat after a subtotal petrosectomy for chronic ear disease. In 2 of the patients, who had 3-month follow-up studies, there was no change in bone conduction thresholds with hearing in the mild to moderate range up to 6 kHz and word recognition scores of 70% and 85% at 80 dB SPL once the Codacs was activated. This improvement is significant compared with their preoperative severe to profound hearing loss. In addition, Barbara and colleagues[15] showed that the Codacs device could also be used for patients with mobile footplates but with severe to profound mixed hearing loss for which the bone conduction threshold is outside the range for an active middle ear implant (>60 dB). A Codacs device was implanted in an ear with a bone conduction threshold in the severe to profound range between 500 and 5 kHz and noted that the pure-tone average was 45 dB 6 weeks postoperatively. In addition, the speech discrimination improved from 20% at activation to 90% at 6-month follow-up. These early studies suggest that the Codacs device has the ability to bridge the gap between active middle ear implants and cochlear implants, thereby providing patients with acoustic hearing for as long as possible.

TOTALLY IMPLANTABLE COCHLEAR IMPLANTS

Cochlear implants use a microphone and processor located external to the ear for capturing sounds. The external positioning places the device at risk for damage during physical activities. In addition, some patients are concerned with the cosmetic appearance of the external device. Over time, these external devices have become less conspicuous. Nevertheless, they are still visible. An early prototype of the totally implantable cochlear implant used a subcutaneous microphone in addition to the external microphone from the external processor of a conventional cochlear implant. This device allowed patients to be without the external device for periods of time. The device was implanted in 3 patients and although patients were able to use their "invisible" hearing, the speech understanding was considerably poorer despite the gradual improvement over time.[16] Nevertheless, all patients used the invisible hearing at various points through the day.

More recently, the Massachusetts Eye and Ear Infirmary and Massachusetts Institute of Technology have collaborated in a proof-of-concept device of a totally implantable cochlear implant. This system also uses a sensor attached to the umbo within the middle ear to detect sound transmitted to the ear canal. Cadaveric studies have shown that an umbo-mounted piezoelectric sensor is able to detect sounds of adequate amplitude across desired frequencies.[17]

Major design requirements for a totally implantable cochlear implant include low power consumption, rechargeable battery, an implantable acoustic sensor that is able to detect sounds from 40 to 90 dB SPL along a similar frequency range to conventional cochlear implants, and an adequate number of spectral electrode channels to balance the benefit of increased speech recognition against the size and power constraints of the device. To minimize the size of the device, an integrated circuit was created that combines auditory sensing, processing, and stimulation into 1 chip.[17]

Future work includes the development of a wireless charging system to rapidly recharge the device throughout the day, as well as the ability to wirelessly transfer data for programming from the audiology team. A further avenue for development involves harnessing in vivo endocochlear electrochemical gradients to serve as a power supply for totally implantable systems, as has been described in guinea pigs.[18]

Pending a clinical trial and US Food and Drug Administration approval, this latest device could afford patients the opportunity to have a nonvisible cochlear implant able to function in almost all situations and environments. This project illustrates the future direction of developing smaller, highly efficient systems through collaboration with scientific specialists.

ROBOTIC COCHLEAR IMPLANTS

Otolaryngology is largely familiar with minimally invasive surgery, including endoscopic sinus surgery, transoral robotic surgery, and more recently endoscopic ear surgery. The concept of fewer and smaller incisions is redefining surgery and has become a paradigm across multiple specialties with proposed benefits such as less pain, shorter recovery, smaller incisions, and shorter hospital stay. One area of investigation is decreasing or eliminating the potential for human surgical error. An ideal, minimally invasive cochlear implant involves creation of a straight tunnel, nearly the size of the electrode, through the mastoid and facial recess to the site of electrode insertion into the cochlea. The margin of error is small given the size of the facial recess, measuring 2.65 ± 0.63 mm in the plane of the round window.[19] Otologic surgeons have impressively shown the ability to perform these surgeries manually with an exceptional safety profile.

Using surgical robots may allow a decrease or elimination of human surgical error in addition to providing a minimally invasive option for some otologic procedures. Nadol and colleagues[20] showed evidence of immediate trauma to the spiral ligament and stria vascularis from cochlear implantation. Robotically controlled placement of an electrode may be able to precisely optimize the correct insertion angle and depth within the scala tympani. Robots currently being used in otolaryngology consist of concurrent, surgeon-initiated movements performed by the robot. As research and development continue, the future is likely to incorporate more fully autonomous robots.[21]

In an effort to automate the cochlear implant drilling, Labadie and colleagues[22] first described the development of a microstereotactic frame combined with a computer-generated automated trajectory to avoid the facial nerve and identify the appropriate location for cochleostomy placement using intraoperative thin-cut temporal bone computed tomography (CT) scans (**Fig. 4**). In their initial cadaveric studies, they showed that the temporal bone drilling of the facial recess with a robot through this microstereotactic frame (as shown in **Fig. 4**B) could be performed to an accuracy of 0.76 ± 0.23 mm.[23] Subsequently, in an initial proof-of-concept study, after the surgeon manually performed a mastoidectomy and facial recess drill-out, a robotic-driven 1-mm sham drill bit (see **Fig. 4**C) was able to be passed through the trajectory determined by the customized microstereotactic frame and avoid the facial nerve in 18 out of 18 patients.[22] They were also able to take this one step further and validate this in pediatric patients, in whom the facial nerve tends to be more lateral and anterior, limiting the view of the round window niche.[24]

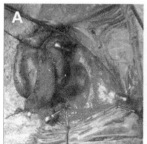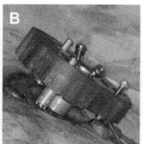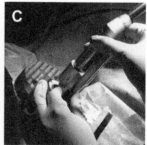

Fig. 4. Setup for a robotic cochlear implant. (*A*) Fiducial markers. Three bone-implanted fiducials are placed along the periphery of the mastoid with extenders with spherical ends. An intraoperative CT scan is obtained with these fiducials in place. (*B*) A custom microstereotactic frame is mounted on the spheres. (*C*) Drill press system attached to the microstereotactic frame. The microstereotactic frame defines the drill path and the drill press controls the linear movement of the drill to a predetermined depth. (*From* Balachandran R, Tsai B, Ramachandra T, et al. Minimally invasive image-guided access for drainage of petrous apex lesions: a case report. Otol Neurotol 2014;35(4):652; with permission.)

In a later study, Labadie and colleagues[25] reported on using customized, patient-specific frames on bone-implanted fiducials (as shown in **Fig. 4**A) for a robot to drill a tunnel along a computer-generated trajectory through the facial recess in 9 patients. In 8 of the 9 patients, the electrode was placed through the drilled tunnel and implanted into the cochlea under direct visualization by raising a tympanomeatal flap. One patient required conversion to the traditional technique because of repeated electrode placement into an air cell. One patient experienced facial nerve paresis thought to be secondary to thermal injury to the nerve. Exploratory surgery on the first postoperative day showed that the bone overlying the nerve was intact.

Using only bone-implanted fiducials without a microstereotactic frame, Caversaccio and colleagues[26] provided a similar description of using a robot to drill a minimally invasive tunnel through the facial recess on the first patient of their 10-patient clinical trial. On conclusion of the robot-performed drilling, a tympanomeatal flap was elevated for visualization of the electrode placement. Postoperative imaging showed expected positioning of the electrode within the scala vestibuli because of noted ossification within the scala tympani.

Despite being more invasive, bone-implanted fiducials have been critical in the development of robotic-assisted cochlear implantation. Relative accuracies of different image-guided systems are shown in **Table 1**. As engineers and scientists work to improve the accuracy of these image-guided systems, it is hoped that one day a fiducial-less registration with the accuracy of bone-implanted fiducials can be achieved so that these robotic systems requiring image guidance can be optimized for better patient outcomes with less invasiveness and fewer complications.

In addition to drilling, robots have been shown to assist with electrode insertion, as shown in **Fig. 5**. Studies have shown that average robotic insertion forces and manual insertion forces by surgeons are similar (0.005 ± 0.014 N for robots and 0.004 ± 0.001 N for surgeons using the Advance Off-Stylet technique), with the surgeons outperforming the robots, but that peak insertion forces between 120° and 200° are much higher with surgeons. There is speculation that decreasing those peak forces would be significant in minimizing trauma-induced damage.[27] Because the inside of the cochlea cannot easily be visualized during the insertion process,

Table 1
Target registration errors for various navigation systems that have been used in otolaryngologic surgery

Image Guidance System	Manufacturer	TRE (mm)	Fiducial
BrainLAB[55]	BrainLAB, Heimstetten, Germany	1.31 ± 0.87	Skin-affixed markers
		2.77 ± 1.64	Laser skin contour
		2.28 ± 0.91	Proprietary headset
InstaTrak[56]	GE Medical Systems, Lawrence, MA	1.97	Skin-affixed markers
StealthStation	Medtronic Surgical Navigation Technologies, Louisville, CO	1.14	Skin-affixed markers[57]
		2.3	Anatomic landmarks[57]
		0.96	Surface merged[57]
		0.49 ± 0.05	Frame with electromagnetic field emitter[58]
Stryker Image Guidance System[59]	Stryker Instruments, Kalamazoo, MI	0.48 ± 0.21	Bone-implanted fiducials

Abbreviation: TRE, target registration error.

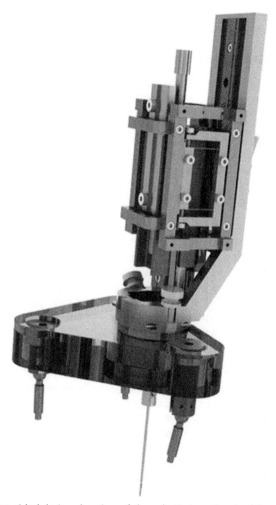

Fig. 5. A computer-aided design drawing of the robotic insertion tool for cochlear implants using the custom microstereotactic table as shown in **Fig. 4**B. (*From* Schurzig D, Webster RJ III, Dietrich M, et al. Force of cochlear implant electrode insertion performed by a robotic insertion tool: comparison of traditional versus advance Off-Stylet techniques. Otol Neurotol 2010;31(8):1210; with permission.)

robots designed to sense insertion forces and modify their trajectory have been developed.[28] Zhang and colleagues[29] took it one step further with a robot that can steer the electrode through the scala tympani to decrease the maximum insertion force by 59.6%.

These pioneers have paved the way for minimally invasive and robotic-assisted cochlear implantation. Possibilities for the future include fully robotic implantation with electrode insertion, which would decrease the invasiveness of the procedure by minimizing the need for a mastoidectomy as well as potentially eliminating human hand unsteadiness, leading to a more atraumatic electrode insertion. This possibility also would make cochlear implantation more accessible to patients who live in areas without well-trained otologic surgeons. Foreseeable issues of implementing robotic surgery may include the patients' confidence and comfort with robots, liability in the setting of a complication, and the potential for deemphasizing the role of surgeons.

ELECTROCOCHLEOGRAPHY AND COCHLEAR IMPLANTATION

In the past decade, there has been significant interest in hearing preservation at the time of cochlear implantation. This interest has resulted in improved surgical technique. However, more importantly, methods to detect hearing preservation and provide real-time feedback at the time of insertion have become a focus of research as surgeons strive to optimize outcomes. Because electrocochleography (ECochG) can provide continuous real-time recordings of physiologic activity of intracochlear tissue and can be detectable even in patients with no measurable audiometric function, intraoperative ECochG using the cochlear implant electrode has recently been explored as a method to detect changes within the cochlea during the time of insertion.[30]

A multi-institutional study of 2 different methods of ECochG, one using the cochlear implant electrode and telemetry and the other using a micrograbber electrode connected to a ground electrode, was able to show gradual increases in ECochG amplitude during the insertion, as expected, although there were instances in which the amplitude remained unchanged or decreased. In addition, electrode manipulation such as packing the round window resulted in large changes in ECochG suggestive of good sensitivity to fluid displacement within the cochlea.[31]

More importantly, ECochG responses have been shown to correlate with postoperative outcomes. Specifically, Fitzpatrick and colleagues[32] showed that the ECochG responses recorded at the round window just before cochlear implant insertion correlated well with postoperative consonant-nucleus-consonant (CNC) scores, even more so than duration of deafness and degree of residual hearing. Although Adunka and colleagues[33] were not able to correlate ECochG responses with residual hearing, many others have shown that ECochG waveforms postoperatively correlate well with audiometric thresholds in patients with residual acoustic hearing.[34,35] Patients with preserved ECochG waveforms were more likely to have preserved hearing and, on average, had 15 dB better audiometric thresholds than those without.[35] In addition, O'Connell and colleagues[36] showed that postoperative ECochG thresholds correlated well with postoperative behavioral thresholds in the lower frequencies. Also, although there was no correlation with intraoperative ECochG thresholds, the difference between these with postoperative audiometric thresholds was significantly better for scala tympani insertions compared with scala vestibule insertions.[36] This finding suggests that, even after implantation, changes in cochlear physiology continue to occur. Nevertheless, the ability to correlate ECochG with postoperative audiometric thresholds suggests that there is potential to provide surgeons with real-time feedback during the insertion. This feedback may allow better, atraumatic insertions into the scala tympani for improved preservation of cochlear structures.

DRUG-ELUTING COCHLEAR IMPLANTS

Cochlear implants function by using an electrode to directly stimulate the auditory nerve fibers within the cochlea. Although traditional cochlear implant candidates have little to no residual hearing, with the increasing popularity of electroacoustic stimulation and excellent hearing outcomes, it is critical to preserve residual hearing in patients that have preoperative measurable low frequency hearing. However, even with preservation of hearing following cochlear implantation, some patients progress to have delayed loss of residual hearing over the upcoming months.[37] This delayed loss has been postulated to arise from localized inflammatory reaction from the trauma associated with implantation as well as from the response to the electrode acting as a foreign body within the cochlea.[38] Nadol and colleagues[20] performed a postmortem analysis of human temporal bones with previous cochlear implants and found that the electrode array commonly had a surrounding fibrous sheath.

Furthermore, O'Leary and colleagues[38] performed a histopathologic analysis of guinea pigs that had undergone hearing preservation cochlear implantation and one of their conclusions was that fibrosis within the cochlea and hearing outcomes may be related. Glucocorticoids are widely used for many inner ear disorders such as sudden sensorineural hearing loss and Meniere disease.[39,40] There have been many investigations regarding systemic and topical administration of glucocorticoids before cochlear implantation. Recently, Kuthubutheen and colleagues[41] performed a randomized controlled trial showing that a preoperative dose of intratympanic steroids given 24 hours before surgery can improve hearing outcomes.

As a result, it is reasonable to conclude that decreasing the amount of inflammation associated with cochlear implantation may result in improved hearing outcomes. This conclusion has led to the development of electrode assemblies containing drug-delivery systems.[42,43] If the delivery system is to remain patent, this could allow chronic infusion of pharmacologic agents within the cochlea. In addition, drug-eluting electrodes using silicone to passively secrete glucocorticoids over a period of time have also been described.[44,45] Drug-eluting cochlear implant arrays may be able to decrease the local inflammation associated with insertion as well as the delayed effects of local reaction to the foreign body within the cochlea.

In the future, pharmacologic-delivering electrodes may continue to be developed and implemented into standard practice as long as the evidence continues to suggest that acute and chronic inflammation within the cochlea can be mediated by medication delivery within the perilymph. Ongoing developments are likely to result in smaller, less traumatic electrodes with drug-eluting properties. Robotic electrode implantation, as described earlier, could also help contribute to minimizing acute inflammation associated with electrode insertion.

OPTICAL COCHLEAR IMPLANT ARRAYS

Cochlear implants are the treatment of choice for patients with bilateral sensorineural hearing loss who do not have meaningful communication ability using alternative methods. The electrodes work by stimulating spiral ganglion nerves by electrical stimulation. The implant arrays contain multiple electrode channels to assist with better-defined sounds; however, it is difficult to isolate the signal to specific neural groups. At the time of surgery, the implant array is blindly inserted within the cochlea, leading to potential suboptimal positioning of the electrodes over ganglion cells within the intended frequency range. This suboptimal positioning leads to interference across electrode channels, contributing to the struggle with speech reception, especially in noisy environments, among cochlear implant recipients.[46]

An avenue to improve implant arrays is to increase the number of electric elements so that more neural groups can be stimulated. The limitation of this technique involves intracochlear spread of the electric signals stimulating surrounding neural groups. Alternative methods to stimulate the cochlea are being investigated to attempt to improve outcomes in cochlear implant patients. The goal is to provide an alternative route of stimulation that would reduce collateral excitation of unintended sound frequencies, reducing artifact and improving patients' hearing. Kallweit and colleagues[47] showed the ability to optically stimulate the cochlea using lasers in guinea pigs. Also, optical electrodes using infrared light to selectively stimulate cochlear neurons in cats have been described.[48] In addition, optogenetics is a technology that has been investigated in animal models and uses light to activate neuronal light-sensitive ion channels in genetically engineered neurons.[49] A potential future outlook for cochlear implants involves arrays composed of multiple light-emitting segments, which could improve on the broad activation associated with the current electrical stimulation pathways, as shown in **Fig. 6**. Further opportunities for improvement in these devices include the ability to precisely program the optical electrode to work with individual variations in cochlear anatomy among patients. Continued research within these technological advancements and demonstration of safety may lead to human clinical applications in the future.

VESTIBULAR IMPLANTS

An additional relevant discussion about the future of implantable auditory devices is the ongoing development of an implantable vestibular prosthesis for bilateral vestibular hypofunction.

The incidence of bilateral vestibular hypofunction is conservatively estimated to be 28 in 100,000 adults according to a data analysis of the 2008 United States National

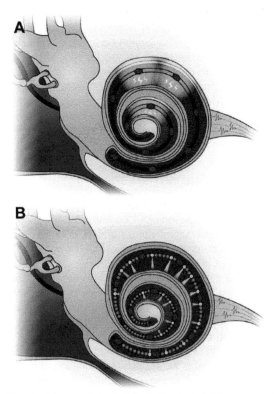

Fig. 6. Current cochlear implants using electrical stimulation (*A*) compared with a proposed optical cochlear implant (*B*). Current cochlear implants currently stimulate broadly, whereas the optical cochlear implant allows finer spatial resolution using focused stimulation with more channels. (*From* Jeschke M, Moser T. Considering optogenetic stimulation for cochlear implants. Hear Res 2015;322:225; with permission.)

Health Interview Survey.[50] These patients experience debilitating balance and visual acuity issues, with an inability to coordinate vestibular sensations with head movement. The current management typically involves vestibular rehabilitation physical therapy.

A vestibular prosthesis has been designed with the goal of providing the neural communication of head rotation to the semicircular canals; however, the design has been limited by the overall size of the implant as well as power consumption.[51] These systems are being designed with gyroscopes to identify head movement and stimulate the appropriate ampullary nerves of the applicable semicircular canals. The electrodes are implanted via a transmastoid approach to implant electrodes near the canal ampullae.[52] More recently, advancements have been made that allow a smaller system that is able to be contained within a typical cochlear implant housing.[53]

Animal studies have shown that the vestibular system can be implanted with stimulating electrodes without causing hearing loss.[52,54] Identified key areas for improvement include decreasing the size and power consumption of the system as well as improving selective nerve stimulation.[52] This area is similar to the issues motivating investigations of alternative stimulation methods associated with cochlear implant arrays. This device further illustrates the focus of future improvements, including smaller, more efficient systems with the ability to selectively target neural groups of interest.

SUMMARY

The future of implantable auditory devices should place an emphasis on making devices accessible to patients while improving hearing and quality of life with maintenance of a desirable safety profile. A common theme among advancements is the development of smaller systems with high efficiency as well as completely implantable systems for the appropriate patient candidates. Smaller systems are often created at the expense of power supply and efficiency; however, advancements have been affected by improvements in microelectronics as well as investigating alternative energy sources. Robotic-assisted or even robotically performed otologic procedures may improve access to surgeries that are typically limited to well-trained otologic surgeons because of the need for accuracy; however, patient comfort, societal impact, and medicolegal ramifications should not be understated. The ongoing and previous successes of auditory technology are the result of collaboration between multiple scientific disciplines. In the future, it is hoped that potential areas for improvement will continue to be identified and translated to clinical research and subsequently to human use.

REFERENCES

1. Jackler RK. The impending end to the stigma of wearing ear devices and its revolutionary implications. Otolo Neurotol 2006;27(3):299–300.

2. Wireless earlens light-driven hearing aid patient instructions. 2017. Available at: https://earlens.com/wp-content/uploads/2018/03/IFU00020vL.pdf. Accessed April 4, 2018.

3. Gantz BJ, Perkins R, Murray M, et al. Light-driven contact hearing aid for broad-spectrum amplification: safety and effectiveness pivotal study. Otol Neurotol 2017;38(3):352–9.

4. Calero D, Paul S, Gesing A, et al. A technical review and evaluation of implantable sensors for hearing devices. Biomed Eng Online 2018;17(1):23.

5. Ko WH, Rui Z, Ping H, et al. Studies of MEMS acoustic sensors as implantable microphones for totally implantable hearing-aid systems. IEEE Trans Biomed Circuits Syst 2009;3(5):277–85.

6. Pfiffner F, Prochazka L, Peus D, et al. A MEMS condenser microphone-based intracochlear acoustic receiver. IEEE Trans Biomed Eng 2017;64(10):2431–8.

7. Park S, Guan X, Kim Y, et al. PVDF-based piezoelectric microphone for sound detection inside the cochlea: toward totally implantable cochlear implants. Trends Hear 2018;22. 2331216518774450.

8. Jang J, Jang JH, Choi H. Biomimetic artificial basilar membranes for next-generation cochlear implants. Adv Healthc Mater 2017;6(21). https://doi.org/10.1002/adhm.201700674.

9. Tona Y, Inaoka T, Ito J, et al. Development of an electrode for the artificial cochlear sensory epithelium. Hear Res 2015;330(Pt A):106–12.

10. Hausler R, Stieger C, Bernhard H, et al. A novel implantable hearing system with direct acoustic cochlear stimulation. Audiol Neurootol 2008;13(4):247–56.

11. Chatzimichalis M, Sim JH, Huber AM. Assessment of a direct acoustic cochlear stimulator. Audiol Neurootol 2012;17(5):299–308.

12. Lenarz T, Zwartenkot JW, Stieger C, et al. Multicenter study with a direct acoustic cochlear implant. Otol Neurotol 2013;34(7):1215–25.

13. Grossohmichen M, Salcher R, Kreipe HH, et al. The Codacs direct acoustic cochlear implant actuator: exploring alternative stimulation sites and their stimulation efficiency. PloS One 2015;10(3):e0119601.

14. Schwab B, Kludt E, Maier H, et al. Subtotal petrosectomy and Codacs: new possibilities in ears with chronic infection. Eur Arch Otorhinolaryngol 2016;273(6):1387–91.

15. Barbara M, Volpini L, Covelli E, et al. Inner ear active hearing device in non-otosclerotic, severe, mixed hearing loss. Otol Neurotol 2016;37(5):520–3.

16. Briggs RJ, Eder HC, Seligman PM, et al. Initial clinical experience with a totally implantable cochlear implant research device. Otol Neurotol 2008;29(2):114–9.

17. Yip M, Jin R, Nakajima HH, et al. A fully-implantable cochlear implant SoC with piezoelectric middle-ear sensor and arbitrary waveform neural stimulation. IEEE J Solid-State Circuits 2015;50(1):214–29.

18. Mercier PP, Lysaght AC, Bandyopadhyay S, et al. Energy extraction from the biologic battery in the inner ear. Nat Biotechnol 2012;30(12):1240–3.

19. Bielamowicz SA, Coker NJ, Jenkins HA, et al. Surgical dimensions of the facial recess in adults and children. Arch Otolaryngol Head Neck Surg 1988;114(5):534–7.

20. Nadol JB Jr, Shiao JY, Burgess BJ, et al. Histopathology of cochlear implants in humans. Ann Otol Rhinol Laryngol 2001;110(9):883–91.

21. Baron S, Eilers H, Munske B, et al. Percutaneous inner-ear access via an image-guided industrial robot system. Proc Inst Mech Eng H 2010;224(5):633–49.

22. Labadie RF, Balachandran R, Mitchell JE, et al. Clinical validation study of percutaneous cochlear access using patient-customized microstereotactic frames. Otol Neurotol 2010;31(1):94–9.

23. Labadie RF, Chodhury P, Cetinkaya E, et al. Minimally invasive, image-guided, facial-recess approach to the middle ear: demonstration of the concept of percutaneous cochlear access in vitro. Otol Neurotol 2005;26(4):557–62.

24. Balachandran R, Reda FA, Noble JH, et al. Minimally invasive image-guided cochlear implantation for pediatric patients: clinical feasibility study. Otolaryngol Head Neck Surg 2014;150(4):631–7.

25. Labadie RF, Balachandran R, Noble JH, et al. Minimally invasive image-guided cochlear implantation surgery: first report of clinical implementation. Laryngoscope 2014;124(8):1915–22.
26. Caversaccio M, Gavaghan K, Wimmer W, et al. Robotic cochlear implantation: surgical procedure and first clinical experience. Acta Otolaryngol 2017;137(4):447–54.
27. Schurzig D, Webster RJ 3rd, Dietrich MS, et al. Force of cochlear implant electrode insertion performed by a robotic insertion tool: comparison of traditional versus Advance Off-Stylet techniques. Otol Neurotol 2010;31(8):1207–10.
28. Schurzig D, Labadie RF, Hussong A, et al. Design of a tool integrating force sensing with automated insertion in cochlear implantation. IEEE ASME Trans Mechatron 2012;17(2):381–9.
29. Zhang J, Wei W, Ding J, et al. Inroads toward robot-assisted cochlear implant surgery using steerable electrode arrays. Otol Neurotol 2010;31(8):1199–206.
30. Choudhury B, Fitzpatrick DC, Buchman CA, et al. Intraoperative round window recordings to acoustic stimuli from cochlear implant patients. Otol Neurotol 2012;33(9):1507–15.
31. Harris MS, Riggs WJ, Koka K, et al. Real-time intracochlear electrocochleography obtained directly through a cochlear implant. Otol Neurotol 2017;38(6):e107–13.
32. Fitzpatrick DC, Campbell AP, Choudhury B, et al. Round window electrocochleography just before cochlear implantation: relationship to word recognition outcomes in adults. Otol Neurotol 2014;35(1):64–71.
33. Adunka OF, Giardina CK, Formeister EJ, et al. Round window electrocochleography before and after cochlear implant electrode insertion. Laryngoscope 2016;126(5):1193–200.
34. Koka K, Saoji AA, Litvak LM. Electrocochleography in cochlear implant recipients with residual hearing: comparison with audiometric thresholds. Ear Hear 2017;38(3):e161–7.
35. Campbell L, Kaicer A, Sly D, et al. Intraoperative real-time cochlear response telemetry predicts hearing preservation in cochlear implantation. Otol Neurotol 2016;37(4):332–8.
36. O'Connell BP, Holder JT, Dwyer RT, et al. Intra- and postoperative electrocochleography may be predictive of final electrode position and postoperative hearing preservation. Front Neurosci 2017;11:291.
37. Barbara M, Mattioni A, Monini S, et al. Delayed loss of residual hearing in Clarion cochlear implant users. J Laryngol Otol 2003;117(11):850–3.
38. O'Leary SJ, Monksfield P, Kel G, et al. Relations between cochlear histopathology and hearing loss in experimental cochlear implantation. Hear Res 2013;298:27–35.
39. Beyea JA, Instrum RS, Agrawal SK, et al. Intratympanic dexamethasone in the treatment of Meniere's disease: a comparison of two techniques. Otol Neurotol 2017;38(6):e173–8.
40. Hara JH, Zhang JA, Gandhi KR, et al. Oral and intratympanic steroid therapy for idiopathic sudden sensorineural hearing loss. Laryngoscope Investig Otolaryngol 2018;3(2):73–7.
41. Kuthubutheen J, Joglekar S, Smith L, et al. The role of preoperative steroids for hearing preservation cochlear implantation: results of a randomized controlled trial. Audiol Neurootol 2017;22(4–5):292–302.
42. Paasche G, Gibson P, Averbeck T, et al. Technical report: modification of a cochlear implant electrode for drug delivery to the inner ear. Otol Neurotol 2003;24(2):222–7.

43. Shepherd RK, Xu J. A multichannel scala tympani electrode array incorporating a drug delivery system for chronic intracochlear infusion. Hear Res 2002;172(1–2): 92–8.
44. Astolfi L, Simoni E, Giarbini N, et al. Cochlear implant and inflammation reaction: safety study of a new steroid-eluting electrode. Hear Res 2016;336:44–52.
45. Farhadi M, Jalessi M, Salehian P, et al. Dexamethasone eluting cochlear implant: histological study in animal model. Cochlear Implants Int 2013;14(1):45–50.
46. Fu QJ, Nogaki G. Noise susceptibility of cochlear implant users: the role of spectral resolution and smearing. J Assoc Res Otolaryngol 2005;6(1):19–27.
47. Kallweit N, Baumhoff P, Krueger A, et al. Optoacoustic effect is responsible for laser-induced cochlear responses. Sci Rep 2016;6:28141.
48. Rajguru SM, Matic AI, Robinson AM, et al. Optical cochlear implants: evaluation of surgical approach and laser parameters in cats. Hear Res 2010;269(1–2): 102–11.
49. Hernandez VH, Gehrt A, Reuter K, et al. Optogenetic stimulation of the auditory pathway. J Clin Invest 2014;124(3):1114–29.
50. Ward BK, Agrawal Y, Hoffman HJ, et al. Prevalence and impact of bilateral vestibular hypofunction: results from the 2008 US National Health Interview Survey. JAMA Otolaryngol Head Neck Surg 2013;139(8):803–10.
51. Della Santina CC, Migliaccio AA, Patel AH. A multichannel semicircular canal neural prosthesis using electrical stimulation to restore 3-D vestibular sensation. IEEE Trans Biomed Eng 2007;54(6 Pt 1):1016–30.
52. Chiang B, Fridman GY, Dai C, et al. Design and performance of a multichannel vestibular prosthesis that restores semicircular canal sensation in rhesus monkey. IEEE Trans Neural Syst Rehabil Eng 2011;19(5):588–98.
53. Hageman KN, Kalayjian ZK, Tejada F, et al. A CMOS neural interface for a multichannel vestibular prosthesis. IEEE Trans Biomed Circuits Syst 2016;10(2): 269–79.
54. Rubinstein JT, Bierer S, Kaneko C, et al. Implantation of the semicircular canals with preservation of hearing and rotational sensitivity: a vestibular neurostimulator suitable for clinical research. Otol Neurotol 2012;33(5):789–96.
55. Schlaier J, Warnat J, Brawanski A. Registration accuracy and practicability of laser-directed surface matching. Comput Aided Surg 2002;7(5):284–90.
56. Fried MP, Kleefield J, Gopal H, et al. Image-guided endoscopic surgery: results of accuracy and performance in a multicenter clinical study using an electromagnetic tracking system. Laryngoscope 1997;107(5):594–601.
57. Pfisterer WK, Papadopoulos S, Drumm DA, et al. Fiducial versus nonfiducial neuronavigation registration assessment and considerations of accuracy. Neurosurgery 2008;62(3 Suppl 1):201–7 [discussion: 207–8].
58. Komune N, Matsushima K, Matsuo S, et al. The accuracy of an electromagnetic navigation system in lateral skull base approaches. Laryngoscope 2017;127(2): 450–9.
59. Pillai P, Sammet S, Ammirati M. Application accuracy of computed tomography-based, image-guided navigation of temporal bone. Neurosurgery 2008;63(4 Suppl 2):326–32 [discussion: 332–23].

Printed and bound by CPI Group (UK) Ltd, Croydon, CR0 4YY

03/10/2024

01040477-0018